PRACTICAL HANDBOOK

of

Sample Size Guidelines for Clinical Trials

IBM-Compatible Version

Jonathan J. Shuster, Ph.D.

Professor of Statistics
University of Florida
Gainesville, Florida

Co-Principal Investigator
Pediatric Oncology Group Statistical Office
St. Louis, Missouri

CRC Press

Boca Raton Ann Arbor London Tokyo

Library of Congress Cataloging-in-Publication Data

Shuster, Jonathan J., 1943-
Practical handbook of sample size guidelines for clinical trials / author, Jonathan J. Shuster. -- IBM-compatible version.
p. cm.
Includes bibliographical references and index.
ISBN 0-8493-4487-5
1. Clinical trials--Statistical methods--Handbooks, manuals, etc.
2. Sampling (Statistics)--Handbooks, manuals, etc. I. Title.
II. Title: Sample size guidelines for clinical trials.
[DNLM: 1. Clinical Trials--methods. 2. Research Design.
3. Statistics. QV 771 S562pa]
R853.S7S55 1992
610'.72--dc20
DNLM/DLC
for Library of Congress 92-49337
CIP

Direct all inquiries to CRC Press, Inc., 2000 Corporate Blvd., N.W., Boca Raton, Florida, 33431.

International Standard Book Number 0-8493-4487-5

Library of Congress Card Number 92-49337

Printed in the United States of America 2 3 4 5 6 7 8 9 0

Printed on acid-free paper

PREFACE

This book is primarily designed as a guide for physicians and biostatisticians working in clinical trials, where the primary objective is survival (or disease-free survival or progression-free survival etc). It will also be useful as a supplement to text material in courses dealing with biostatistics.

To project patient needs of a trial, the physician needs to provide "planning parameters". These include endpoints (eg 3 Year survival); minimum difference the trial is to be sensitive to (eg 50% control vs 65% experimental); patient accrual rate (eg 55 patients per year are expected to be accrued); precision measures ("ALPHA"=probability of falsely concluding experimental therapy has efficacy given that it has none: typically .05) ("POWER"=probability of correctly concluding the experimental therapy has efficacy when the minimum difference is as above: typically .8 or .9 depending on the field); and anticipated rate of patient losses for non-study related reasons called "LOSSES TO FOLLOW-UP".

This handbook is organized into three chapters, an appendix, and program disk. CHAPTER 1, "*How to Use the Sample Size Program*", is designed for users who simply want to know how many patients they need. This section is therefore a "Cookbook" approach, including a worksheet for obtaining the appropriate sample size for the trial. CHAPTER 2, "*Design and Analysis of Randomized Clinical Trials*", is a non-technical discussion of the major elements of such trials. This section may be helpful for the user wishing to write a clinical protocol or a clinical research grant. A blueprint for protocol construction is included. CHAPTER 3, "*Derivation of the Statistical Results*", contains a heuristic derivation of the statistical methods presented in CHAPTER 2. One full year of Calculus-based Mathematical Statistics is sufficient background to understand the material in CHAPTER 3. In addition, this chapter contains some simple results on multiple comparisons and stratified analysis (in non-technical language). APPENDIX 1 contains a fairly detailed review of Mathematical Statistics, thereby making the text self-contained with respect to CHAPTER 3.

Summary of what you need to read:

1. Cookbook: Give me the sample size needed. (CHAPTER 1)
2. Clinicians: Help me write my Research Protocol. (CHAPTERS 1 and 2. For a discussion of "losses to

follow-up'', the reader might also consult Section 3.10 of CHAPTER 3. If the study has more than two treatments, see Section 3.12 of CHAPTER 3. Although that Section is far more technical than CHAPTER 2, most clinical investigators should be able to follow the main ideas. If after reading CHAPTER 2, ''stratification'' is contemplated, see Section 3.13 of CHAPTER 3.)

3. Biostatisticians: Entire text material.

   Extensions and Limitations: While the major scope of this Handbook is for two treatment randomized trials, CHAPTER 3 (Section 3.12) does contain methods for the design and analysis of trials involving three or more treatments. This Handbook is limited in scope to therapeutic comparisons involving survival (or disease-free survival or progression-free survival, etc) as the primary endpoint. Analysis of prognostic factors are not discussed.

NOTE: In any Clinical Trial, it is in everyone's best interest that a team of researchers be assembled at the planning stage. This team should consist of clinical researchers, a biostatistician, and computer scientists. Laboratory researchers are often important members of the team.

THE AUTHOR

Jonathan J. Shuster, Ph.D., is currently a Professor in the Department of Statistics, University of Florida, Gainesville, Florida. He serves as Co-Principal Investigator of the Statistical Coordinating Center of the Pediatric Oncology Group, which at any time has at least 75 active multi-center clinical trials in childhood cancer. Apart from cancer, he has participated in major collaborative projects in Ophthalmology and Urology. He has published over 80 articles in methodologic research and in medical applications. His major statistical research interests include the design and analysis of clinical trials and of large epidemiologic studies.

Dr. Shuster has served on numerous NIH Study Sections including the Epidemiology and Disease Control Study Section #1 (1986—90). He served as Chair of that Study Section for the 1989—1990 fiscal year. It is largely through service on these study sections that Dr. Shuster recognized the need for this book.

In addition to his research efforts, Dr. Shuster has been active in teaching. He has taught service statistics courses to students in the health sciences, as well as elementary, intermediate, and advanced courses in statistics.

Dr. Shuster received his Ph.D. degree from McGill University, Montreal, Canada in 1969. Since then, he has been at the University of Florida. As of the spring of 1990, he had received nearly $10 million in grants, mostly from the National Institutes of Health.

The author wishes to express his appreciation to many kind friends who directly contributed to this project, most notably to Dr. Jim Boyett, to Dr. Dick Scheaffer, and especially to Dr. Jeff Krischer.

This book is dedicated to Isobel and Samuel Shuster, parents of the author, on the occasion of their golden wedding anniversary.

TABLE OF CONTENTS

Chapter 1

HOW TO USE THE SAMPLE SIZE PROGRAM

Introduction

It is vital that a clinical trial has a reasonable chance of achieving its objectives. Small negative studies could be harmful, as they might not have had adequate power to find important differences. Researchers might falsely conclude from the completed trial that a new therapy lacks efficacy. Freiman et al (1978) reviewed a large number of published negative studies and concluded that the vast majority were not adequately sensitive to clinically meaningful differences. To avoid this problem, clinical trials must be well designed, and must have sufficient numbers of patients to answer the study question.

In order to use the sample size program, the user must supply several values called parameters. The worksheet, Figure 2, will be helpful. Before getting too formal, let us have a glance at a "Statistical Consideration" of a research protocol. At first, it probably will look quite technical, but we shall unravel the details.

STATISTICAL CONSIDERATION

"Historically, the Institute has been able to accrue 125 patients per year with newly diagnosed X-disease. Based on our prior studies, the three year survival rate is expected to be about 60% on the standard therapy (or control therapy). In order to detect a 15% improvement under the experimental therapy (three year survival of 75%), at "alpha"=.05 (one-sided) and 80% "power", a sample size of 204, half randomly assigned to each treatment, will be needed. This calculation assumes exponential survival with all patients followed to death or termination point of the study. Allowing for a 10% loss to follow-up, a figure consistent with past history, a revised sample size of 227 (1.8 years of accrual) is needed. Patients will be followed until death, loss to follow-up, or the completion of the study (up to 4.8 years). The logrank test will be used to make the treatment comparison."

1.1 Identification of Parameters:

(1) Annual Accrual

125 Patients per year (Input in program)

(2) Minimum Planned Follow-up: At how many years will the key survival comparison be made?

3 years (Input in program)

(3) Expected Accrual thru Minimum Follow-up

125 X 3=375 (Calculated by program)

(4) PCONT=Planning value for survival thru the minimum follow-up period (In this case 3 years) under the CONTROL treatment.

.6 (ie 60%) (Input in program)

(5) DEL=Planning value of improvement under the experimental treatment at the endpoint (ie at three years in this case.)

.15 (ie 15%) (Input in program)

(6) ALPHA=Chance of falsely concluding experimental therapy is superior to the control, when in fact it is equivalent to the control. In most studies, a value of .05 (ie 5%) is used. There is no special reason to pick this value other than standardization. For further discussion, see Chapter 2, especially as to one-sided versus two-sided tests. See also the footnote at the conclusion of the chapter.

.05 (ie 5%) (Input from menu in program)

(7) POWER=Chance of correctly concluding that the experimental therapy is superior to the control, when in fact the planning values (4) and (5) are correct. The most common values for power are 80% and 90% depending on the field. This is discussed further in Chapter 2 and in the footnote at the end of this chapter.

.80 (ie 80%) (Input from menu in program)

(8) FACT (for factor). This asks the following question. Consider a typical day before and after the endpoint. A value of FACT is the ratio of the instantaneous death rate after the endpoint to that before the endpoint. The exponential distribution implies a value of 1.0. If you consider patients cured after three years, you would use a value of 0. However, the program can be used for intermediate situations. For example, you might consider that the typical day more than three years out carries half the risk of the typical day less than three years out. In that case, you would use a value of FACT=.5 (or 50%).

A sample size value for BIN(binomial) is also provided in the program. This gives the sample size required if you only looked the "Binary" event of surviving three years or not surviving three years. The comparison would ignore time of death and all data collected after the patient had made it to the three year point. This comparison is distinct from the logrank test and carries a different sample size. This alternate and less powerful test is discussed in Chapter 2 under the name "Kaplan-Meier." If you "browse" through the program, you will note that for many situations, the FACT=.00 and FACT=BIN sample size requirements are very close. When FACT=.00, no deaths are expected after the endpoint.

1.0 (ie 100%) (Exponential) (Input in program)

(9) LFU (Losses to Follow-up)=fraction of patients expected to be lost to competing causes (eg quitting or failing for causes unrelated to the study endpoint).

.10 (ie 10%) (Input in Program)

SUMMARY OF INPUT

(1) ANNUAL ACCRUAL=125

(2) ENDPOINT(YEARS)=3

(4) PCONT=.60

(5) DEL=.15

(6) ALPHA=.05 (One-sided) (enter 4 to menu ?)

(7) POWER=.80 (enter 6 to menu ?)

(8) FACT=1.0

(9) LFU=.10

To obtain the sample size, you need simply provide the above entries in response to the questions posed by the program.

The output is:

Initial Sample Size= 204 (Without LFU)

Initial accrual duration=1.632 years

Final Sample Size=227 (allows 10% LFU)

Final accrual duration=1.816 years

Report after 4.816 years

(Parallel binomial sample sizes are 235(initial) 262 with LFU.)

*** Footnote on one-sided vs two-sided tests. In situations where you wish to compare two treatments, neither of which can be viewed as a control, you should run a two-sided test. Basically, you proceed exactly as above but replace the value of ALPHA by ALPHA/2. If the above study consisted of two experimental therapies, we would use ALPHA=.025. (menu choice 3) For the 45% vs 60% comparison, we would use PCONT=.45 and DEL=.15, with FACT=1.0. This would require 282 patients. For the 60% vs 75% comparison, we would use PCONT=.60 and DEL=.15 with FACT=1.0. This would require 250 patients. To be safe, we take the larger of these two numbers, 282. Allowing for 10% loss to follow-up, the final sample size would be 313 (2.5 years of accrual).

*** Further Reading. The sample size results of this **handbook** are similar to those of Schoenfeld (1981), Rubinstein et al. (1981), and especially Lachin (1981, where his equations (25) and (26) are employed). Another interesting method is due to Halpern and Brown (1987), who offer a computer program which can simulate the properties of the logrank statistic under any survival distributions provided by the user.

Finally, a method of Sposto and Sather(1985) is useful in some applications. That method yields similar results to those of this handbook.

REFERENCES

1. **Freiman, J. A., Chalmers, T. C., Smith H., and Keubler, R.,** The importance of beta, the type II error and sample size in the design and interpretation of the randomized controlled trial, *N. Engl. J. Med.*, 299, 690, 1987.
2. **Halpern, J. and Brown, B. W.,** Designing clinical trials with arbitrary specification of survival functions for the log rank or generalized Wilcoxon test, *Control. Clin. Trials,* 8, 177, 1987.
3. **Lachin, J.,** Introduction to sample size determination and power analysis for clincial trials. *Control. Clin. Trials,* 2, 93, 1981.
4. **Rubinstein, L. V., Gail, M. H., and Santner, T. J.,** Planning the duration of a comparitive clinical trial with loss to follow-up and a period of continued observation, *J. Chron. Dis.*, 34, 469, 1981.
5. **Schoenfeld, D.,** The asymptotic properties of nonparametric tests for comparing survival distributions, *Biometrika,* 68, 316, 1981.
6. **Sposto, R. and Sather, H. N.,** Determining the duration of comparitive clinical trials while allowing for cure, *J. Chron. Dis.*, 38, 683, 1985.

FIGURE 1: Use of Sample Size Program

A. IBM Version (DOS)

1. To run from floppy: Put disk in floppy drive. Type A:crcssiz

2. To put on hard disk in directory CRC (Drive C).

```
MD\CRC
CD\CRC
COPY a:*.*
```

   Back up by putting a formatted disk in drive A

   COPY CRC*.* a: (Store in place remote from computer.)

3. To run from hard disk (after completing 2 above)

```
CD\CRC
CRCSSIZ
```

4. Respond to each Question by providing requested data and pressing the ENTER key. See Figure 2 for requested data.

B. Macintosh Version

Copy from floppy to appropriate folder
Double Click on CRCSSIZ icon

Back-up by copying file from folder to new floppy.
(Store in place remote from computer.)

Respond to each Question by providing requested data and pressing the ENTER key. See Figure 2 for requested data.

NB: This program was compiled using Microsoft QuickBASIC 4.0(IBM) and QuickBASIC 1.0(MAC).

FIGURE 2: Worksheet For Sample Size Determination

One-Sided Studies
50% assigned to each treatment.

(1)	Expected Annual Accrual	_____ (Patients) ENTER
(2)	Endpoint (? Year Survival) Minimum Planned Follow-up	_____ (Years) ENTER
(3)	Expected Accrual thru Minimum Follow-up (Program Calculates this)	_____ (1)X(2)
(4)	PCONT (Control Planning Survival Probability to Endpoint)	_____ (Decimal) ENTER
(5)	DEL (Planned improvement in Survival to Endpoint under Experimental Treatment)	_____ (Decimal) ENTER
(6)	ALPHA=Probability of concluding experimental therapy superior when it is equivalent to control (menu choice)	_____ (Decimal) ENTER
(7)	Power=Probability of correctly concluding experimental therapy superior when DEL is as in (5) (menu)	_____ (Decimal) ENTER
(8)	FACT=Ratio of instantaneous death rate after the endpoint to that before the endpoint	_____ (Decimal) ENTER
(9)	Estimated Fraction to be Lost to Follow-up	_____ (Decimal) ENTER
	OUTPUT OF PROGRAM	
(10)	Identify Initial Sample Size (Ignores losses to follow-up)	_____ (Patients)
(11)	Final Sample Size (10) divided by (9)	_____ (Patients)
(12)	Accrual Period (11) divided by (1)	_____ (Years)
(13)	Total Study Duration (2)+(12)	_____ (Years)

FIGURE 3. Modifications of Figure 2

1: FOR TWO-SIDED TESTS

(A) Replace ALPHA by ALPHA/2 in (6).

(B) Replace PCONT by the lower of the two planning survival probabilities in (4)

(C) Replace DEL by the difference between the two planning survival probabilities in (5).

(D) Proceed as in Figure 2. (You may have to do this twice if the planning survival probability is known for one of the experimental therapies while the other is planned at from DEL worse to DEL better. If this is the case, do both calculations and use the larger of the two sample sizes.)

2: FOR UNEQUAL PATIENT ALLOCATION (ie not a 50-50 randomization) (Valid for allocations from 33% to 67%)

(A) Find the sample size as if the allocation was 50-50 using FIGURE 2 (and FIGURE 3-1 if needed)

(B) Adjust as Follows

Allocation 2:1(67%) or 1:2(33%),Multiply result in (A) by 9/8

Allocation 3:2(60%) or 2:3(40%),Multiply result in (A) by 25/24

Allocation X:Y,Multiply result in (A) by (X+Y)(X+Y)/(4XY)

Note that this sample size is always higher than a 50-50 allocation.

Chapter 2

DESIGN AND ANALYSIS OF RANDOMIZED CLINICAL TRIALS

This chapter is a concise non-technical introduction to the design and analysis of randomized clinical trials. For more detail, at a non-technical level, the reader is referred to the following excellent references: Pocock (1983), Buyse et al (1984), and Meinert (1986). While the methods of this volume apply to very specific types of trials, they are in fact applicable to the majority of major definitive trials run today. We shall discuss clinical trials in a more general framework, but restrict our analytic considerations to randomized trials.

We shall discuss the trials under each of their four basic steps:

1. Formulate a therapeutic research question.
2. Design a trial to answer this question.
3. Conduct the trial as planned.
4. Analyze the data and report the results.

2.1 Formulation of the Therapeutic Question

This part of the trial is more medical than statistical. The question might be, for example, "Can Beta-Blocker X improve survival of newly diagnosed myocardial infarction patients over that of the standard Beta-Blocker Y?" This is the type of question which can form the starting point of a clinical trial. Note that there are two competing therapies proposed for this trial. While this book is devoted to two treatment trials, Section 3.12 provides extended use for more complicated questions involving three or more competing therapies.

Note that the research question is very loosely worded at this point. There will be considerable work to convert this question into a truly testable hypothesis.

2.1.1. One-Sided vs Two-Sided Question

An important component of your research question is whether your question is "one-sided" or "two-sided". The following discussion will help make this determination.

When you conduct a clinical trial, you will usually put on trial one of the following statements

1. One-Sided Statement: The new (test) therapy is superior to the standard; or

2. One of the two therapies is superior to the other, but you have no vested interest as to which.

Sample One-Sided Questions

Drug companies, developing a new drug, are generally interested in one-sided questions. Their product may only be marketable if they can prove beyond a reasonable doubt that their product is superior to the standard. The competing therapies have asymmetrical interest.

Again, if any scientific researcher is considering the efficacy of adding a toxic agent to a standard regimen, and comparing this to the standard regimen alone, a one-sided question results. After the study is over, one would use the new therapy only if it proved to be significantly better than the standard. Whether the efficacies were not significantly different or the toxic agent had significantly reduced the efficacy, one would make the management decision not to use this toxic agent for future patients.

Sample Two-Sided Questions

There may be two standard therapies that are in widespread use, but no one really knows which is superior. The scientific issue here is simply, which is the better therapy? Interest is symmetric.

In some diseases, there may be no known effective therapy. One might wish to test two new experimental therapies. Here too, a two-sided question is clear.

One-sided questions need fewer subjects than two-sided questions of equal precision. The "Zone of proof beyond a reasonable doubt" is concentrated in the zone where the test treatment outperforms the control treatment. The two-sided question must create two such zones, one corresponding to superiority of each treatment. Consequently, the region of superiority of each given treatment must be smaller in the two-sided question corresponding to the one-sided question of the same precision.

The one-sided vs. two-sided question must be spelled out in advance as a vital part of the research question. Clear-cut rationale for asymmetric interest must be given. In point of fact, most trials conducted in the medical school environment should be two-sided, unless there is a compelling reason for asymmetry.

2.2 Design of the Clinical Trial

In order to conduct a valid clinical trial, it is vital to develop a complete plan for its conduct. A manual of operations, called a "Protocol", should be written with the following elements:

A. Objectives of the Study (What you hope to accomplish.)

B. Background Information (Literature review of prior therapy and outcome. Include your own experience as well.)

C. Rationale (Why you feel you have good prospects to achieve your objectives.)

D. Patient Eligibility (A Precise definition as to who can participate in the trial.)

E. Treatment Plans (Full description of how patients will be treated under each competing therapy. This must include contingency plans for complications.)

F. Off-Study Requirements (Full description of events that place the patient off study. For example, patient may go off study at time of recurrence of disease, allergic reaction to the drug, or death.)

G. Data Submission Requirements (This describes the schedule of follow-up, the medical tests required and their timing, and the description and timing of the data form submission.)

H. Statistical Consideration. (This describes the actual design, including the endpoint of the study, whether stratification and randomization will be used, plans for interim and final analysis, and sample size projections. If the study is a "masked design", this is also discussed in this Section.)

I. Study Monitoring (A committee called the Data Safety and Monitoring Committee should be listed along with their meeting schedules and responsibilities.)

J. Appendix (This should include blank copies of all data forms and the informed consent form. Instructions on forms completion should also be included.)

K. Database Documentation (While this may not be a formal part of the protocol, it is a critical element of the design. A protocol cannot be compromised by turnover in computer staff.)

This author was once sent a computer tape of a trial completed some six years earlier, in order to re-analyze the data. Unfortunately, the senders lacked documentation of the data. Despite our best efforts, we could not crack the code with enough confidence to complete any analysis.

2.2.1 Statistical Considerations

In planning a trial, there are a number of issues that need to be considered in (H) above. First, the eligibility conditions define the "Target Population". This is the hypothetical pool of past, present, and future patients with well defined characteristics. Note that the actual patients who participate in the study are considered to be a representative sample from this target population. Our ultimate conclusions will be directed to the target population not to the sample. Of course, we use the sample data to make an inference about this target population. Such inferences are subject to sampling error, since only a portion of the target population has been sampled. This is much like the use of voter surveys to project election results.

Answers to the following question are needed to formulate the statistical consideration.

What is the single primary variable upon which the major comparison will be based?

It is essential to pin down a primary variable up front. If this is not specified, the data may be analyzed in a wide variety of ways, leading to investigator selection bias. Each analysis carries a sampling error, and hence the more analyses one performs, the greater the cumulative error effect. To control this, a primary single analysis should be specified. Others can be done, but as strictly secondary analysis. Example primary variables might be three year remission, five year survival, two year peak intra-ocular pressure below 23 mm hg, etc.

As mentioned in the Introduction, there are two types of primary variables considered in this Handbook. The first type is "Censored Survival Data". Time is measured from entry onto the study until failure, termination of the study, or loss to follow-up. The last occurs if the patient exercises his or her option to quit the study. The only survival information available are (1) the time from entry to last follow-up and (2) the patient status at last follow-up. The data are censored (or more precisely, right censored), since for survivors, we do not know their true survival times, although we do know that they survived at least a given number of days (eg 655+ days). The second type of data in which these sample size tables can be used is binary data (yes/no). For example, a study on operative deaths (whether or not the patient died during surgery), is not concerned with time of death, but only whether or not the patient survived the surgical procedure. Unlike the censored survival situation, follow-up is short and equivalent for all patients. In a censored survival study, involving a three year patient accrual phase plus a two year minimum follow-up (a five year total study), patients have a potential follow-up of from two to five years. The risk of a study death among earlier entries is higher than that among later entries, since the early entries are at risk longer. This needs to be taken into account in the analysis. The operative death problem is quite different. The only data used in that analysis is whether or not the patient survived surgery.

Will the study be randomized?

This is a controversial topic. Let us suppose that you plan to compare two therapies. You may have considerable experience with one of the therapies (the "control" or "standard") and little experience on the other (the "experimental" or "test"). You may ask, "Why not simply recruit patients to the experimental regimen and compare these to the existing control patients?" This is called an "Historical Control Study". There are both advantages and disadvantages of such a strategy. Historical control studies often require fewer patients than randomized studies, and hence can often be completed in less time and at less cost than concurrently controlled studies. Unfortunately, however, historical control studies cannot be viewed as definitive scientific evidence about the relative merits of the competing therapies. You cannot adequately attribute differences (or lack of differences) in outcome with differences in efficacy. Subtle changes in any of the following can hopelessly confound the results of an historical control trial: Changes in referral pattern, changes in personnel, changes in diagnostic techniques, changes in concomitant care, changes in public awareness programs, etc. In addition, the trial may have been motivated by disappointing results under the standard therapy. Disappointment is more likely when the sampling error under the historical control is negative than it would be if the sampling error is positive. In other words, suppose the true success rate is 60% under the standard. A 50% observed success rate in your sample of 50 historical patients could provide greater motivation to conduct a study than a 70% observed success rate.

One advantage of historical control studies, not often mentioned in publications, is the issue of gaining informed consent. It is very difficult to approach a patient in order to gain consent for randomization. Uncertainty in a physician can undermine the confidence of the patient. However, in truth, the same uncertainty is generally present in the historical control study, although it is often downplayed.

Finally, historical control studies are fully justified if the historical control success rate is virtually zero. In such cases, you are unwilling to subject patients to a hopeless therapy. Even here, however, there is no unanimous agreement among scientists. For example, in 1986, randomized studies were conducted in AIDS patients, using a control known to offer no hope for survival. Surprisingly, there was a strong moral argument for the randomization. Since only a limited number of patients were approved for initial testing of new agents, a randomized design could treat as many patients as a non-randomized design. Further, by careful interim comparison of treatment vs. control patients, the randomized study offers the best way to study non-fatal events. For additional information on randomized vs. historical controls, see Zelen (1983), Shuster et al. (1985), Pocock (1983), Gehan (1978 and 1982), Peto et al. (1976), Diehl and Perry(1986), and Dupont (1985). These articles present all sides of the issues.

In summary, a randomized study is recommended very strongly, except perhaps when the historical success rate is near zero. However, if you consider a randomized study and determine that the required sample size is too large, an historical control study might be considered. Prior to doing so, however, the possibility of running a randomized study with additional institutions should be seriously considered.

Note: Randomization is a more complex topic than one might at first believe. It is important that the investigator cannot predict what therapy the next patient will be assigned. The purpose of randomization is threefold. First, it prevents unconscious bias in treatment assignment as compared to non- randomized assignment. Second, the framework of statistical analysis relies on randomization. Finally, a properly set up randomization procedure offers an audit trail of treatment assignments. This protects the investigator if the results of a study are questioned by a review group or by journal editors.

Randomization Methods

Some randomization techniques are discussed in Pocock (1983, Chapter 5). Figure 4 presents a table of randomized treatment assignments, based on "simple randomization". Each successive entry is an independent flip of an unbiased coin (50% probability of heads). Heads represents treatment 1, while tails represents treatment 2. Figure 5 represents an alternate design, with "random length permuted blocks". The following is the mechanism for Figure 5. First, a balanced coin is flipped. If the coin is heads, then we generate a random "word" consisting of three 1's and three 2's. Each of the possible 20 words consisting of three 1's and three 2's has an equal chance of occurring. If the coin lands tails, then we generate a random word consisting of two 1's and two 2's. Each of the following six equally likely words is drawn: 1122, 1212, 1221, 2112, 2121, 2211 This procedure is repeated, until the figure is completed. These figures provide the serial assignment of treatments for successive patients.

Simple randomization (Figure 4) is very simple to employ, but may lead to rather substantial differences in the number of patients assigned to each therapy. To illustrate, after 813 randomizations in Figure 4, there are 443 patients assigned to Treatment #1 and 370 assigned to treatment #2, for a net difference of 73 patients. This is the peak difference over the 1200 patient assignments. The random length permuted blocks procedure keeps the numbers well balanced throughout the study, while it is quite unpredictable to the investigator, especially if the exact mechanism of randomization is masked. Randomization is discussed further under stratification and institutional balancing below.

Will the study be stratified?

Are there key "risk factors" that need to be balanced "prospectively" or "retrospectively"? There is always concern that a randomized design will place a disproportionate number of poor risk patients on one of the treatments. If one has historical information about such risk factors, they might be planned for in two ways. First, we may wish to stratify the trial prospectively. That is, we shall define patient subgroups according to the risk factors, and essentially run independent trials within each subgroup. Using random length permuted blocks within each subgroup, we can maintain good balance of the treatments across each stratum. This is a good design feature, but it comes at a price. Over stratification can reduce the precision. Peto et al. (1976) estimate that the effective sample size of the study is reduced by one for each stratum you create, as compared to the luckily perfectly balanced randomized trial. For example, a trial stratified on age group (4 levels), sex (2 levels), smoking history (3 levels), and serum cholesterol (3 levels) would create 4 X 2 X 3 X 3 = 72 strata. Clearly, a poorly designed study could be so heavily stratified that there would be very few patients in any one stratum. The purpose of stratification is to compare like patients with like patients. However, stratification limits the possibility of comparison, as the following example illustrates. Suppose that there are 100 patients, 50 in stratum 1 and 50 in stratum 2. Suppose that 50 are assigned to each treatment. The un-stratified design allows 50 treatment #1 patients each to be compared to 50 treatment #2 patients (2500 comparisons). The stratified design eliminates half of these, namely patients in different strata and different treatments. Clearly, there is a trade-off. We recommend only very limited stratification, based on important proven risk factors, be made.

The second method to deal with stratification is to adjust for the risk factors retrospectively in the analysis. This method is discussed in CHAPTER 3.13. The reader is further referred to Peto et al. (1977). No within-stratum balancing is done, but imbalances are corrected for in the analysis.

If the study is a multi-center study, will institutional balancing be used?

When conducting a multi-institutional study, especially if it is conducted by a large number of institutions, each with a relatively small number of patients, one should consider balancing the randomization within institutions. While it seems that this might create too many strata, especially if the study is also stratified according to risk factors, a method called "Marginal Balancing" can be used to avert this problem. Basically, marginal balancing, as discussed in Shuster et al. (1985), works as follows. Assign the patient according to prior assignments for the institution and stratum as follows:

Priority #1: Check how many patients have been assigned to each treatment at this institution. If the difference between the number of assignments exceeds the maximum allowable margin, (say 2), assign the treatment that has been assigned less often at that institution. For example, if at X-Hospital, 7 patients are on Treatment #1 and 4 patients are on Treatment #2, and the maximum allowable margin for randomization is 2, the next patient at this institution must receive Treatment #2.

Priority #2: Applies only if Priority #1 has not forced a treatment assignment. For the patient's stratum, check the number of patients assigned to each treatment. If the difference exceeds the maximum allowable margin for randomization, assign the less used treatment. (Note that the stratum maximum margin need not match that of the institution.)

Priority #3: Applies only if Priorities #1 and #2 have not forced a treatment assignment. Assign treatment according to the next unused entry on the random length permuted block assignment sheet. (For example, Figure 5.)

Bookkeeping: After each patient assignment, it is necessary to update the number of patients assigned to each therapy by institution and stratum. In addition, the assignment should be recorded on the random length permuted block assignment sheet by crossing off the first available entry matching the assigned treatment. This will be the next entry if Priority #3 applies.

Marginal balancing keeps institutions and strata balanced. It also keeps the overall study balanced because of the permuted blocks. One of the advantages of marginal balancing is that the study can be analyzed as if it was a single institutional study. In other words, one can ignore the stratification effect of institution in the analysis. This is especially important in studies conducted by a large number of institutions with a large number of strata. In practice, the "error" one makes in treating the study as a single institutional study is in the conservative direction. That is, there will be a slight tendency to underestimate the significance of the differences between the treatments (overestimate the "P-values"). However, this error is rarely of practical significance.

Marginal balancing is also important for non-statistical reasons in studies where some institutions contribute small numbers of patients. Each institution should gain experience on both therapies. Without institutional balancing, there is more than a 12% chance that an institution contributing four patients will place all four on the same treatment.

If the study is multi-institutional, will centralized randomization be employed?

Centralized randomization is strongly recommended for all multi-center trials. Clearly, if marginal balancing is used, a central office must have up-to-the-minute information on all prior treatment assignments. There are more important considerations, however. The integrity of the study is best insured through centralized randomization. No patient can get onto the study without contact with the central office. Eligibility can be verified by standardized criteria prior to acceptance of the patient. Without centralized randomization, the study is open to the possibility that early failures may never be placed on the study. Individual investigators may overlook the important task of forwarding the information on such patients to the central office. With centralized registration and randomization, patients must be put on study before starting treatment. Registration and randomization need not be done at the same time. Some studies will have both treatments identical for the first 6-12 weeks, followed by a divergence. All participants should be registered at the time of treatment start, but a callback for randomization should occur at the time when the treatments diverge. This callback will in fact improve the precision of the comparison, since the major comparison will be based on outcomes after the divergence point. Failures before the divergence point are not part of the study question, although they are vital to the estimation of the efficacy of each therapy. The treatment differences must occur after the divergence point, but the overall success rate of each therapy is measured from the start of treatment. You have the luxury of using all patients (regardless of assigned therapy) to assess the efficacy of the therapy from its starting point to the divergence point.

Will the study be masked (blinded)?

It is a good experimental technique to mask the identity of the treatment from both the patient and the investigator. (The more common term is blinded, but as one with experience in ophthalmic trials, your author considers that designation is a bit short sighted.) Masking is an especially important consideration if (1) patient psychological factors may be involved, (2) the response measurements involve subjective judgement on the part of the physician or the patient, or (3) the treatment can be put in a masked form, ethically and logistically. Contra-indications for masking include possible discomfort to the control patient; the need for the physician to perform expensive and/or painful medical tests to monitor one of the treatments and its side-effects; and the ability to mask the therapy. It would be unethical to perform sham surgery on a patient in order to mask the true procedure.

Some masking is better than no masking. For example, if it is unethical to mask the treating physician, it might be possible to have the critical observations made by a colleague who is indeed masked as to the treatment identity. A vital consideration in masked studies is that the master code, indicating who got each treatment, be securely maintained. More than one masked study has failed because the master code was lost! If such a loss occurs, nothing can be done to recover.

What methods of analysis will be used?

This will be discussed further in Section 2.4. However, the statistical section must spell out the exact statistical details as to what methodology will be used.

This needs to be specified in the protocol, as a protection to the investigators. Journal reviewers can sometimes criticize a study on the basis that it was not analyzed according to the design of the study. The best protection against this contingency is to submit a copy of the protocol with the manuscript. Often, the protocol itself undergoes peer review, and hence is strong support for your analysis.

What patients will be included in the analysis?

In most studies, there will be some severe violations of the protocol, often for reasons beyond the control of the investigators. The question one might pose is, "Will the major comparison be based on all compliant patients, or on all eligible patients?" There is now fairly unanimous agreement that the most convincing scientific analysis is based on all eligible patients. Once a patient is deemed to meet the entry requirements, that patient is included in the major analysis, whether or not the patient complies with the assigned protocol. This is often called "The Intent to Treat Principle". Many journals have published policy that the major analysis must consist of all patients who meet the eligibility conditions, whether or not they comply with the protocol. Two important editorials supporting this point are

Zelen (1983) and Simon and Wittes (1985). As soon as subjective judgement is allowed to enter the picture, the potential for bias arises. Other analysis can be done as secondary evidence. However, severe bias can be induced by eliminating non-compliant patients. Compliance can have a strange relationship to treatment, apart from merely a disproportionate number of non-compliers within the two treatment groups. Non-compliers on one treatment may be at increased risk, while non-compliers on the other treatment may be at decreased risk. The "Intent to Treat Principle" also implies that patients are analyzed on the treatment to which they were assigned, even if they actually received the other therapy! This may seem to be invalid at first glance, but it is the only way to prevent bias. The argument is that the Intent to Treat Principle closely resembles the real world application of the treatment. Poor compliance to a protocol will adversely affect its success. It is vital to keep track of compliance, but the major analysis should not utilize compliance. For additional detail on this topic, see Shuster et al (1985), Simon and Wittes (1985), and Haynes and Dante (1987).

What are the plans for interim analysis?

When conducting a long term trial, there is considerable motivation to look at the results to date to see if the question can be answered early. Such a plan for example led to the early closure of the Multi-Institutional Osteosarcoma Trial of Link et al. (1986). That protocol specified times for interim analysis as well as conditions which would lead to early termination of the study. It needs to be pointed out that the decision to close a study early should be based on very compelling evidence. Generally speaking, the more interim analyses that are conducted, the greater the risk of false positive results. If interim analyses are to be conducted, they should be conducted at a very small P-value as compared to a one-time final analysis. This can be put into a formal statistical methodology called "Group Sequential Methods" or in a more informal way, where the critical P-value is a small fraction of the final planning P-value. (Eg .005 for interim analysis vs .05 for the final planned analysis.) For more information on this topic see Armitage (1975), O'Brien and Fleming (1979) and Tsiatis and Rosner (1985).

In any case, the protocol should spell out exactly when interim analyses will be conducted, and how decisions based on interim analyses will be made. If an interim analysis does in fact suggest that the study be terminated, the decision should not be made until the data have been reviewed carefully by the "Data Safety and Monitoring Committee". See Section 2.2 (I) discussed earlier.

2.3 Conduct of the Trial

Once the trial is opened to patient accrual, there are many elements which are required to ensure that the trial meets its objectives. Each institution must obtain annual approval from its Institutional Review Board (IRB) in order to register patients on the study. In order to place any patient on the trial, informed written consent must be obtained. The risks and benefits of the competing therapies must be explained as well as the objectives of the study. If the trial is randomized, the patient should know this before the treatment is assigned. There are some pre-consent randomization designs. See Zelen (1979 and 1982), Smith (1983), and Fletcher (1985) for more details. Such designs are highly controversial as these references point out. The vast majority of studies assume randomization after consent, unless the patient is incapable of giving informed consent, Abramson et al. (1985).

The patient becomes part of the trial as soon as consent is obtained. Further, once treatment is assigned, the patient is a part of that treatment group, regardless of whether or not the patient complies with the therapy. The investigator is ethically bound to follow the therapy as prescribed in the protocol, unless there is overwhelming evidence that violating the protocol is in the patient's best health interest. The patient assumes no legal commitment to follow the protocol, but does so in the spirit of physician-patient relationship.

Data Submission

It is the responsibility of each investigator to fully comply with all data submission requirements of the trial. Even the world's most outstanding statistician is limited by the quality and quantity of data submitted by the investigators. Even small amounts of missing data can bias a study.

Interim Analysis

A well -written protocol has provisions for interim analysis. However, it is important that while the trial is accruing patients, this information should be restricted to the Data Safety and Monitoring Committee. Investigators should not see interim treatment comparisons while patient accrual is ongoing. The committee is charged with the responsibility of determining if randomization remains ethical. With open reporting, selection bias could result from individualized analysis on the part of the investigators.

In some situations, it may be important to mask the treatment comparisons until all patients have completed therapy. For example, suppose that Treatment A consists of two years of Beta-Blocker X, while Treatment B consists of two years of Beta-Blocker Y, from the time of myocardial infarction. If an unblinded interim analysis shows a trend in favor of B, some investigators may want to switch their A patients to B. This could compromise the entire trial. The decision to switch or not switch should be in the hands of the Data Safety and Monitoring Committee, not the individual investigator.

Protocol Amendments

Once a protocol is actively accruing patients, amendments should be resisted. However, even the most carefully written protocols are not immune to unexpected results. For example, one might encounter toxicities, that had not occurred in pilot studies. Counter measures would have to be written into the protocol. If the counter measure has efficacy implications on one or both treatments, then the amendment may have the effect of forcing the investigators to start the accrual process over. The patients already accrued would not be used in the comparison of the treatments. Each amendment has to be sent back to the IRBs for approval. In addition, the Statistical Consideration and Consent Form will need modifications to incorporate these amendments. Amendments must be handled with as much precision as the original protocol.

2.4 Analysis and Reporting of the Trial

Upon completion of the accrual phase and minimum projected follow-up on all patients, the final analysis phase begins. The first step is to acquire all possible delinquent and missing information. Next, the analysis is completed as prescribed in the Statistical Consideration. Finally, the results of the trial are submitted for publication in a refereed medical journal.

2.4.1. Crucial Elements

The analysis described in the statistical section must be employed in the analysis. The sample size calculation only applies to the statistical methods detailed in the protocol.

Definition of P-value: The methodology of the statistical consideration provides an ordering of the possible outcomes in terms of how well they support a difference between the treatments (one-sided or two sided as specified in the design.) The P-value is interpreted as follows: Suppose that you repeated this study in another universe where the treatments were in fact equivalent. What is the maximum probability of observing evidence of a difference in this repetition that is as least as convincing as that observed in the actual trial? (The answer is the P-Value.) For example, suppose that the observed success rate of the test treatment was 46/84 while that in the control treatment was 34/81. The statement, which we shall discuss in more detail below is, "P = .05 one-sided." That is, if we repeated our protocol in a population where the success rates are equal, then there is at most a 5% chance of observing a difference of 12.8% or more in favor of the test treatment. (46/84-34/81 = .128=12.8%).

Methods of Analysis of Clinical Trial Data

We shall discuss three methods of analysis of clinical trial data. These include Sections 2.4.2, Binomial Comparison; 2.4.3, Kaplan-Meier Comparison, and 2.4.4, Logrank Comparison.

2.4.2 Binomial Comparison

The Binomial Comparison is applied to trials where the outcome is binary: Success or Failure. The following properties must be satisfied, at least conceptually, in order to apply this methodology:

P1: Trials are "INDEPENDENT". That is, the outcome of a given patient is not influenced by the outcome of any other patient. This methodology should not be used for matched studies, since the outcome of one patient will have more predictive value on the matched patient than it would on any other patient.

P2: The "Success Probability" within a given treatment is the same from patient to patient. That is, without knowing the patient characteristics in advance, the probabilities of success in the first, second, third, ... patients assigned to the given treatment are equal. For censored survival studies where patients enter serially and where the study is analyzed at a fixed point in time, this assumption is violated. Early entries are at risk for a longer period than later entries, and hence, have lower success rates than later entries. Of course, the success rate of each treatment need not be the same.

2.4.2.1 Large Sample Methodology

Let N1=Sample Size for the Standard or Control Therapy

S1=Number of Successes in the Control Sample

F1=Number of Failures in the Control Sample

P1=S1/N1=Fraction of Successes in the Control Sample.

Let N2=Sample Size for the Test Therapy

S2=Number of Successes in the Test Sample

F2=Number of Failures in the Test Sample

P2=S2/N2=Fraction of Successes in the Test Sample.

The difference in Success rates is P2-P1. We also need a quantity called the "Estimated Variance of P2-P1", denoted by:

$$V=\{P1(1-P1)/N1\}+\{P2(1-P2)/N2\}$$

The test statistic for which a decision about the therapies is based is:

$$Z=(P2-P1)/SE$$

where

$$SE=SQRT(V) \qquad \text{(SQRT=Square Root)}$$

The approximate "P-value" associated with Z is obtained from FIGURE 6 for one-sided comparisons and from FIGURE 7 for two- sided comparisons. The intuitive interpretation of the P-value is given in Section 2.4.1.

2.4.2.2 Confidence Intervals

Another more descriptive way to report the above information is via a CONFIDENCE INTERVAL. A "One-Sided Confidence Interval" is reported for DEL, the true target population difference in success rates, as:

$$DEL > P2-P1-W\ SE$$

where W is selected from Figure 8 according to the desired confidence. The intuitive interpretation of the Confidence Interval is given below Figure 8.

A "Two-Sided Confidence Interval" is reported as:

$$P2\text{-}P1+W\ SE > DEL > (P2\text{-}P1)\text{-}W\ SE$$

where W is selected from Figure 9 according to the desired confidence. The intuitive interpretation of the Confidence Interval is given below Figure 9.

2.4.2.3 Numerical Example (Test)

Suppose that the Control therapy had N1=81 patients of whom S1=34 were successes and F1=47 were failures. We have P1=34/81=0.420. Suppose further that the Test therapy had N2=84 patients of whom S2=46 were successes and F2=38 were failures. Hence, P2=46/84=0.548.

To calculate V, note that 1-P1=1-.420=.580 and 1-P2=1-.548=.452.

$$V=\{(.420)(.580)/81\}+\{(.548)(.452)/84\}=\{.2463/81\}+\{.2477/84\}=0.00304+0.00295=.00599$$

$$SE=SQRT(V)=.0774$$

and

$$P2\text{-}P1=.548\text{-}.420=.128$$

Hence,

$$Z=.128/.0774=1.653$$

From Figure 6, this translates to a P-Value of slightly less than 0.05, for a one-sided test. Had this been a two-sided study, we see from Figure 7 that the two-sided P-value is slightly less than 0.10. Finally, if the Experimental and Test labels had been reversed so that the Experimental group had 34 successes in 81 patients while the Control group had 46 successes in 84 patients, the One-Sided P-Value would have been approximately 0.95.

2.4.2.4 Numerical Example (One-Sided Confidence Interval)

If one was to construct a 95% One-Sided Confidence Interval for DEL, the target difference in success rates, one would employ FIGURE 8:

$$DEL > .128-1.645\{.0774\}=.128-.127=.01$$

That is, DEL> .01 with 95% confidence.

Notice that the value of Zero, the point of equal efficacy, lies just outside the confidence interval. (Had the P-value been greater than 0.05, Zero would have appeared within the confidence interval. The two-sided confidence interval will illustrate this.)

2.4.2.5 Numerical Example (Two-Sided Confidence Interval)

Had this been a two-sided question, a 95% two-sided confidence interval would be obtained from Figure 9 as follows:

$$.128 + 1.96\{.0774\} > DEL > .128-1.96\{.0774\}$$

That is .28 >DEL > -.02 with 95% confidence.

Had this been a two-sided experiment, the outcome would not have achieved statistical significance at the conventional .05 level. However, we are highly confident that the Test treatment ranges from trivially inferior to vastly superior. The value in the confidence region most favorable to the control treatment represents only a 2% advantage to the control. The confidence interval allows a management decision to prefer the test treatment for future patients, despite the fact that conventional significance of the two-sided trial was not achieved. The P-Value alone does not allow this type of management logic.

2.4.2.6 Small Sample Methodology

In order to apply the Large Sample Methodology, the following rules of thumb are often used:

Each of the following four quantities are greater than 5.0:

N1(S1 + S2)/(N1 + N2) = "Expected Successes for Control"

N1(F1 + F2)/(N1 + N2) = "Expected Failures for Control"

N2(S1 + S2)/(N1 + N2) = "Expected Successes for Test "

N2(F1 + F2)/(N1 + N2) = "Expected Failures for Test "

The term "Expected" refers to the idealized distribution of the actual patient results to the two groups, where the success rate would be the same in both treatment groups.There is nothing magic about the number 5.0. However, the approximations seem to be "adequate" at this number of patients.

Generally speaking, if a randomized clinical trial is designed to be sensitive to clinically relevant differences, the approximations made for large samples will be valid. However, in very small trials with low power, exact methods are needed. The two most widely used methods are Fisher's Exact Test and the Exact Unconditional Z Test. We shall discuss these briefly. For more detail, the reader should consult Armitage (1971), Suissa and Shuster (1985), and Shuster (1988).

Fisher's Exact Test

In the numerical example above, imagine that we have a deck of cards, distributed as follows: 80 Cards are labeled SUCCESS and 85 Cards are labeled FAILURE, for a total of 165 cards. Now suppose that we randomly distribute the cards to two players called Control and Test (81 to Control and 84 to Test). What is the probability of distributing 46 or more successes to the Test player? In other words, if we repeated the experiment on a different target population, where in fact the control and test therapies were equivalent, and if we happened to again get a total of 80 Successes and 85 Failures, what is the likelihood of obtaining evidence at least as convincing as that observed in favor of the test therapy? The answer is P=.068. (The approximation had P=.05 one-sided)

Note that this is not a true P-value, since the additional proviso is made that in the replication of the experiment, you must match the total number of successes with that observed (80). We call such a P-Value "an Exact Conditional P-Value" to remind us that it was calculated under an added artificial condition.

A two-sided analogue of Fisher's Exact Test is also possible. The observed difference in success rates was P2-P1=.128.

If we had seen 44 successes in 81 controls and 36 successes in 84 test (keeping the total successes at 80), then the difference in success rates would have been .115; while the difference between 45/81 vs 35/84 is .139. On a two-sided basis, if the test group is dealt either (A) 46 or more successes or (B) 35 or fewer successes, the evidence in favor of a difference would be at least as strong as that observed (.128).The probability that either (A) or (B) occurs in redeals is:

P=.120 (Conditional) vs P=.10 (2-sided approx.)

The P-value requires the same condition in the replication of matching total successes to that observed. Thus, this is not a true P-value, but rather a conditional one.

Exact Unconditional P-Value

The Exact Unconditional Z-test works as follows. The observed Z value was 1.653. What is the probability that if we had 81 independent success/failure observations for control and 84 success/failure observations for test, with the success rate identical for both control and test, that we would observe a Z-value of at least 1.653? The answer may depend on the value of that common success rate. The exact unconditional Z-test maximizes this probability over all possible identical values for the success rates (from 0 to 1). According to the definition, this yields the P-value. A microcomputer program (including hardware requirements), to perform the calculations is described in Shuster (1988). The one-sided version considers values above the observed Z of 1.653 in favor of the test treatment, while the two-sided version considers values above the observed value of 1.653 in favor of either treatment.

The exact unconditional P-values are .057 (vs approximation of .05 one-sided) and .108 (vs approximation of .10 two-sided). These agree remarkably well.

As Suissa and Shuster (1985) point out, the Exact Unconditional Z-Test generally outperforms Fisher's Exact Test. (Requires fewer patients for trials.)

2.4.3 Kaplan-Meier Comparison (Large Sample)

The Kaplan-Meier (1958) methodology is designed to estimate the probability of surviving for a given number of years, utilizing "Censored Survival Data". Unlike the Binomial methods above, the Kaplan-Meier technique recognizes the possibility that patients' times at risk will be unequal. However, the Kaplan-Meier technique makes the very important assumption that the prognosis of a patient who withdraws from the study is the same as that of a patient of the same "age" who remains on the study. This means for example, that the prognosis of a patient who was lost to follow-up after 6 months on the test therapy is the same after the six month point as that of a patient still on the test therapy at six months. It is therefore clear that in many studies, the validity of the Kaplan-Meier method rests heavily on obtaining virtually complete follow-up on all patients. Note that the above assumption is reasonable for patients whose follow-up is short, but current. For example, it is reasonable to assume that if a patient entered the study six months before it was to be analyzed he/she has the same outlook post six months as that of a patient who entered the study on the first day the study opened, four years prior to the analysis.

For each treatment, the Kaplan-Meier curve provides an estimate of the true probability of surviving at least T-days. The true probability represents the hypothetical target population of all past, present, and future patients who meet the eligibility conditions of the study. The estimate is based on the sample of patients assigned to the given treatment. It is subject to sampling error, since the actual sample assigned to the treatment is assumed to be a conceptual random sample from the target population. It also could be subject to selection biases, if the sample of patients cannot be viewed as a conceptual random sample from the target population. A good example where selection bias can occur, is where there is selective participation by some institutions in a multi-center trial. For example, institution X agrees only to place their advanced patients on a study.

2.4.3.1 Assumptions Underlying the Kaplan-Meier Curve

P1. All observations are "INDEPENDENT". That is, the outcome of a given patient is not influenced by that of another.

P2. Given the treatment assignment, the survival probability distribution of each patient over time is the same from trial to trial. In other words, patient prognosis on the test treatment is the same for early entries in the trial as later entries. The same holds true within the control treatment.

P3. The loss to follow-up rate is very small. Otherwise, we assume that patient losses are not in any way influenced by the patient's prognosis. Failure of this assumption is especially serious if one of the therapies is more toxic, leading to vastly differing withdrawal rates between the treatments.

Comment: Withdrawals for toxicity probably violate this assumption. It is therefore vital to keep track of study losses to toxicity.

2.4.3.2 Calculation of the Kaplan-Meier Curve

The Kaplan-Meier curve starts at DAY 0 at a value of 1.00(100%). On each succeeding day, we compute the value from the preceding day as follows:

Let R=Number of patients left at risk on that day(At Risk)

F=Number of patient failures on that day (Deaths)

$$KM = KM\text{ (on previous day) } X\ (R-F) / R \qquad (1)$$

The estimate is easily justified intuitively as follows. The estimate is built on a day-to-day basis, using the data for each day. To survive 100 days, a patient has to survive day 1, day 2,...., day 100. The logical estimate of the probability of surviving a given day, assuming that the patient was alive at the start of that day, is (R-F)/R, the ratio of the number of patients who survived that day to the number at risk on that day. The Kaplan-Meier estimate for day 100 is simply the product of the (R-F)/R values for days 1,2,3,...,100. An analogy to successive taxes will further motivate the multiplication. Imagine that you wish to send $1000 to a relative in Angola. The money is routed as follows. First it goes to Canada, which extracts 1%. Next, it goes to Cuba, which takes 13% of the balance. Finally, it goes to Angola, which charges 16% of what is left. We see that 99% survives the first taxation; of that, 87% survives the second taxation; and of that, 84% survives the final levy.

Surviving Gift=$1000X.99X.87X.84=$723.49

1. Canada: 1% of $1000.00 tax ; 99% of $1000=$990 survives

2. Cuba : 13% of $990.00 tax ; 87% of $ 990=$861.30 survives

3. Angola: 16% of $861.30 tax:84% of $861.30=$723.49 survives.

Note that the KM value in (1) stays the same as the previous day, unless at least one failure occurs. We shall demonstrate the curve concept for the Control Treatment (See Figures 10 and 11).

2.4.3.3 Numerical Example: See Figures 10 and 11.

Control Kaplan-Meier Curve

On Day 1, F=2 and R=186 and hence (R-F)/R=184/186.

On Day 2, only 184 patients are at risk, two having been lost on day 1. For Day 2, F=1 and R=184 and hence (R-F)/R=183/184.

On Days 3-6, no failures occurred and hence (R-F)/R=1.000.

On Day 7, F=1 and R=183, and hence (R-F)/R=182/183.

On Days 8-11, no failures occurred and hence (R-F)/R=1.000.

On Day 12, no failure occurred, but one survivor had only 12 days of follow-up. Here too, F=0 and hence (R-F)/R=1.000.

On Days 13-15, no failures occurred and hence (R-F)/R=1.000.

On Day 16, F=1 and R=181, and hence (R-F)/R=180/181.

This process continues to day 3454.

On Day 1, KM=184/186=.98925.

On Day 2, KM=.98925X183/184=.98387.

On Days 3-6, KM stays at .98387, but on Day 7,

KM=.98387X182/183=.97850

On Days 8-15, KM stays at .97850, but on Day 16

KM=.97850X181/182=.97309

This process continues to day 3454.

Wouldn't a computer be nice? There are many excellent programs for both mainframe computers and micro-computers.

2.4.3.4 Standard Error

A second important quantity relative to the Kaplan-Meier Curve is the "Standard Error". This latter quantity is used to obtain confidence intervals for fixed term survival as well as for comparison of fixed term survival for two competing treatments. There are several forms of the standard error, but the most convenient is due to Peto et al (1977, Statistical Note 6).

For a given day,

SE=KM SQRT{(1-KM)/RX} (2)

With KM as in (1) above. RX is the number at risk at the start of the following day. [Some users replace RX by the value of R from (1). However, in nearly all cases, the alternate SE is virtually identical to that of (2).]

One-sided and two-sided approximate confidence intervals can be obtained (using W from Figures 8 and 9 respectively) for a single fixed term survival as: True Survival >KM-(W SE) One-Sided Upper (Figure 8)

True Survival <KM+(W SE)	One-Sided Upper (Figure 8)
True survival <KM+(W SE)	One-Sided (Lower Figure 8)
KM-(W SE) <True Survival <KM+(W SE)	Two-Sided (Figure 9)

From Figure 11, at three years, we see that KM=51.6%(.516) for the Control Group. RX=91, the number at risk at the start of Year 4, ie the next day. Note that there was no failure in the control group (Figure 10) at day 365*3=1095. Hence, R may be taken as the number at risk at the start of year 4 (Interval 3-4 Years), that is, R=91. In this case, the alternate SE is the same as that computed in (2).

SE= .516 SQRT {(1-.516)/91

= .516 SQRT (.484/91)

= .516 SQRT (.005319)

= .516 X .0729

= .038 (or 3.8% as per Figure 11)

A One-sided 95% confidence interval for three-year survival is:

True control 3-year survival>.516-1.645X.038=.453

A Two-sided 95% confidence interval for three-year survival is:

.516-1.96X.038<True Control 3-year survival<.516+1.96X.038

that is between .442 and .590.

2.4.3.5 The Kaplan-Meier Comparison of Two Treatments

For the desired fixed term (eg 3 years), the following quantities are obtained: Control Group: KM1 and SE1, the Kaplan-Meier estimate and Standard Error at the desired time. Test Group: KM2 and SE2, the Kaplan-Meier estimate and Standard Error at the desired time.

Calculation of approximate P-value:

Let

$$Z = (KM2-KM1)/SQRT(SE1^2 + SE2^2) \tag{3}$$

Utilize Figure 6 (One-sided) or Figure 7 (Two-sided) to obtain the P-value.

In the numerical example of Figures 10 and 11, taken at three years,

KM1=.516 SE1=.038

KM2=.589 SE2=.036

$Z=(.589-.516)/SQRT(.038^2 + .036^2)$

$=.073/SQRT(.001444+.001296)$

=.073/SQRT(.002740)

=.073/.0523

=1.39

From Figure 6, the approximate P-value is .085, one-sided. (Had this been a two-sided comparison, the approximate P-value would have been .17. See Figure 7.)

2.4.3.6 Confidence Intervals for Difference in Fixed-Term Survival

Confidence Intervals for the difference in Fixed Term Survival can also be constructed. As in the Binomial example, they can be important in management decisions.

KM2-KM1 = Estimated difference in True survival at prescribed times (Eg 3 years).

SED=SQRT($SE1^2$ +$SE2^2$) is the Standard Error of this difference

A one-sided confidence interval is obtained using W from Figure 8 as:

True difference in fixed survival>(KM2-KM1)- W SED

A two-sided confidence interval is obtained using W from Figure 9 as:

(KM2-KM1)- W SED < True Difference < (KM2-KM1) + W SED

A one-sided 95% confidence interval in the numerical example of Figures 10 and 11 at three years is: (See calculation of Z above)

True difference in three year survival>(.073)-1.645X.0523

>-.013

The corresponding two-sided 95% confidence interval at three years is:

$$-.030=.073-1.96 \times .0523 < \text{True Difference} < .073 + 1.96 \times .0523 = .176$$

As in the binomial case, the practical implication of the confidence interval over that of the P-value alone is clear. With high confidence, we can state that the test treatment has from a 3.0% disadvantage to a 17.6% advantage in three year survival, when compared to that of the control. If disadvantages of the order of 3% are not considered to be clinically significant, then the test therapy is preferred, even though conventional significance at $P<.05$ was not achieved.

2.4.4 Logrank Test

By far the most common method of comparing treatments in censored survival experiments is via the logrank test. Justification for the name is somewhat technical. (Interested readers might refer to Section 5 of Peto and Peto (1972) for the rationale behind the name). The major difference between the Kaplan-Meier and Logrank tests concern the question which each asks. The Kaplan-Meier comparison asks if the survival probabilities differ at one and only one pre-specified point in time (eg 5 Years). The logrank test asks if the survival curves differ. In other words, the logrank comparison looks at the entire available spectrum of time and attempts to distinguish between the treatments on the basis of overall performance in terms of survival.

For each day, starting the clock at randomization, the data used is:

N1=Number of patients on the control therapy at risk at the start of that day.

F1=Number of control therapy patients who fail on that day.

N2=Number of patients on the test therapy at risk at the start of that day.

F2=Number of test therapy patients who fail on that day.

If we are asking the question: Are the therapies equivalent in terms of survival, we would expect that given the total number of failures on that day, that they would tend to be distributed to treatment groups in proportion to the number at risk in that group. We calculate

$$E1=N1(F1+F2)/(N1+N2) \text{ and } E2=N2(F1+F2)/(N1+N2)$$

The Logrank test looks at F1 vs. E1 and F2 vs. E2 across days. Suppose that when one adds across days, the F1 total vastly exceeds the E1 total. That is, the control therapy has many more failures than one would expect for equivalent therapy. One would infer that the hypothesis of equivalence was in doubt, and accept the hypothesis that the test therapy was superior. Conversely, fewer than expected failures on the control therapy would lead to inferred superiority of the control therapy.

In order to formalize this into a statistical test, a quantity, V is calculated for each day as follows. Suppose a deck of (N1+N2) cards has (F1+F2) failures. If we shuffle this deck and assign N1 to player "Control" and N2 to player "Test", we would expect on average E1 failures to be assigned to "Control" and E2 to "Test". The quantity V is the "Variance" in the number assigned, that is the AVERAGE SQUARED DIFFERENCE between the randomly dealt assignment and the EXPECTED ASSIGNMENT.

If N1+N2>1 then

$$V=N1N2(F1+F2)(N1+N2-F1-F2)/\{(N1+N2)(N1+N2)(N1+N2-1)\}$$

If N1+N2 = 1 then V=0.

The logrank statistic is defined as:

$$Z=\{Sum(F1)-Sum(E1)\}/SQRT\{Sum(V)\} ,$$

where Sum is taken over each day for which patients are on study.

An approximate P-value is obtained from Figure 6 for one-sided tests and from Figure 7 for two-sided tests.

2.4.4.1 Important Observations with Respect to the Logrank Test

Prior to studying a particular example, we note the following:

1. Days on which no failure occurs make no contribution to Z. On such days, F1=0, E1=0 (since F1+F2=0), and V=0. Hence, the sum can be restricted to days on which failures occur.

2. If either N1=0 (only test patients left on that day) or N2=0 (only control patients left on that day), no contribution to Z is made. Clearly, if N1=0, then F1=0, E1=0, and V=0. If N2=0 then clearly the number of test therapy failures on the day (F2) is zero. This further implies from the above formulas that E1=F1 and V=0. The contribution to the Sum(F1) is counterbalanced by that to Sum(E1). Hence, such days have no impact on either the numerator or denominator of Z.

3. On many studies, only one failure will occur on any given day. If this occurs,

$$V=N1N2/\{(N1+N2)(N1+N2)\}=E1E2. \text{ (One Failure)}$$

4. E1+E2=F1+F2. (See formulas).

5. Provided that relatively few failures occur on any given day, an excellent approximation for Sum(V) is

$$\text{Sum(V)} \doteq \text{Sum(E1)Sum(E2)}/\{\text{Sum(E1)+Sum(E2)}\}$$

$$\doteq \text{Sum(E1)Sum(E2)/(Total Number of Deaths)}$$

2.4.4.2 Numerical Example

Suppose that the control group survival (in days) is:

20,49+,122,245,301,332+,355+,378,398,402+,455,467+

while the experimental group survival is:

28+,122,255+,301+,344+,366,388+,409+,444+,477+,500,553+,

the survival in a randomized study of 24 patients. Only values followed by + indicate surviving patients.

The following table is a worksheet for the logrank test. Only days on which failures occur are included.

Day	N1	F1	N2	F2	E1	E2	V
20	12	1	12	0	.500	.500	.250
122	10	1	11	1	.952	1.048	.474
245	9	1	10	0	.474	.526	.249
301	8	1	9	0	.471	.529	.249
366	5	0	7	1	.417	.583	.243
378	5	1	6	0	.455	.545	.248
398	4	1	5	0	.444	.556	.247
455	2	1	3	0	.400	.600	.240
500	0	0	2	1	.000	1.000	.000
Sum		7		3	4.113	5.887	2.200

Z=(7-4.113)/SQRT(2.200)=2.887/1.483=1.95

From Figure 6, this translates to a one-sided P=0.026.

Sample calculation for day 122 — As can be seen from the data, there were 10 Control and 11 Test Patients alive at the start of Day 122. (Of the 12 controls, two did not reach day 122. One died at day 20 and another is alive but has only reached day 49.) (Of the 12 test patients, one is alive but has only reached day 28.) As can be seen from the data, one patient in each group failed on Day 122, and hence. F1=1 and F2=1. From the formulas for E1 and E2:

E1=N1(F1+F2)/(N1+N2)= (10X2)/21=20/21=.952

E2=N2(F1+F2)/(N1+N2)= (11X2)/21=22/21=1.048

V=N1N2(F1+F2)(N1+N2-F1-F2)/{(N1+N2)(N1+N2)(N1+N2-1)}

=(10X11X2X19)/(21X21X20)=4180/8820=.474

All other entries in the above table had only one failure on the day and hence for THOSE DAYS ONLY,E1=Proportion of patients on Control, E2=Proportion of patients on test, and V=E1E2.

2.4.4.3 Footnotes to Numerical Example and the Logrank Test

1. The approximation of Sum(V) in the above example is

$$\text{Sum(V)} \doteq \text{Sum(E1)Sum(E2)}/\{\text{Sum(E1)+Sum(E2)}\}$$

$$\doteq 4.113\text{X}5.887/(4.113+5.887) = 2.421$$

Had we used this approximation, we would have obtained:

$$Z \doteq 2.887/\text{SQRT}(2.421)=2.887/1.556=1.86$$

instead of Z=1.95.

2. For large trials, despite the simplicity of the ideas, a computer would be most helpful in completing the analysis.

3. The validity of the approximate P-values depends on the accuracy of the "Normal Approximations". Generally speaking, for most applications, the approximations are acceptable if Sum(E1) and Sum(E2) both are five or more. The above example would be a borderline case.

As a check on the validity of the above one-sided P-value, we ran a small simulation study as follows. For each of 250 allocations, 12 patients were randomly reallocated to either the "Control" and 12 to the "Test" group. Using the same survival data, 4 of these reallocations had Z at least 1.95 in favor of the "Test" group. If there really was no target difference between the therapies, then any hypothetical allocation of the 24 patients into groups of 12 would be equally likely. Thus, of the 251 allocations (including the actual one), 5 (including the actual one) were 1.95 or higher. This yields a P-Value of about .020, one-sided. While as pointed out in Shuster and Boyett (1979) that this is a legitimate Exact "Conditional" P-value, it should be viewed as an approximation to complete enumeration of the 2.7 million possible reallocations of the 24 patients into two groups of 12.

A review of the definition of P-Values will be needed to grasp the next paragraph. See Section 2.4.1 (Crucial Elements).

Conditional P-values, as mentioned in the section on Fisher's Exact Test, are similar to other P-values, except that they impose artificial restrictions on the replication process used in our definition of P-Value. For this simulation study, the restrictions are that the same 24 outcomes are obtained, and the actual replicated treatment assignment is randomly picked from the 251 assignments (250 from simulation study plus the actual observed assignment.)

4. For trials involving more than one treatment, see section 3.12 of Chapter 3. Note that "Z sub ALPHA" and "Z sub BETA" are the upper 100ALPHA% and upper 100BETA% point of the Standard Normal Distribution (Figure 6).

5. If the trial is stratified, the analysis can be conducted as per CHAPTER 3, Section 3.13. This is a non-technical section, but the notation is slightly different.

Corresponding Values for Each Stratum

	CHAPTER 2	**CHAPTER 3 (Section 3.13)**
Failures on Treatment #1	Sum(F1)	O
Expected Failures on Treatment #1	Sum(E1)	X
Variance	Sum(V)	V

2.4.4.4 Proportional Hazards and the Logrank Test

While the logrank test is valid for testing the equality of two survival curves, it has large sample optimality properties, see Peto and Peto (1972), for the "proportional hazards" situation defined below. The sample size methods of this Handbook are computed under this model.

Proportional Hazards Model Assumption

Under a Proportional Hazards Model, we assume that the hazard ratio, the ratio of instantaneous death rates (Control:test), does not depend on the time on test. To make the assumption concrete, suppose that the probability that an individual alive 6 months post randomization has a 1/1000 chance of dying on the next day under the test therapy and a 2/1000 chance of dying on the next day under the control therapy. Considering a day as an instant, the ratio of instantaneous death rates is:

$$(2/1000)/(1/1000)=2.0 \text{ at 6 months.}$$

While the treatment specific instantaneous death rates are allowed to change over time in the proportional hazards model, the ratio is assumed to be constant over time. If the instantaneous death rates for the test group is 1/3000 at 2 years, we assume it is 2/3000 (double) at 3 years in the control group, since otherwise, the ratio at 6 months would not be the same as that at 2 years.

This assumption is only used in calculating the sample size. Failure of this assumption does not render the logrank test invalid as a device to compare the equality of two survival distributions.

REFERENCES

1. **Abramson, N.S., Meisel J.D., and Safer P.,** Deferred consent: a new approach for resuscitation on comatose patients. *JAMA*, 255, 2466,1986.
2. **Armitage, P.,** *Statistical Methods in Medical Research*, Blackwell Scientific, Oxford, England,1971.
3. **Armitage, P.,** *Sequential Medical Trials*, Blackwell Scientific, Oxford, England,1975.
4. **Buyse, M.E., Staquet, M.J., and Sylvester, R.J.,** *Cancer Clinical Trials: Methods and Practice*. Oxford University Press, England, 1984.
5. **Diehl, L.F., and Perry, D.J.,** A comparison of randomized concurrent controls with matched historical controls: are historical controls valid?, *J Clin. Oncol.*, 4, 114, 1986.

6. **Dupont, W.,** Randomized vs. historical clinical trials: are the benefits worth the cost?, *Am. J. Epidemiol.*, 122, 940, 1985.

7. **Fletcher R. H.,** Clinical trials, randomized consent and estimation (letter and response), *J. Chron. Dis.*, 37, 953, 1984.

8. **Gehan, E. A.,** Comparative clinical trials with historical controls, *Biomedicine*, 28 (Special issue), 13, 1978.

9. **Gehan, E. A.,** Randomized or historical control groups in cancer clinical trials: are historical controls valid?, *J. Clin. Oncol.*, 4, 1024, 1986.

10. **Haynes, R. B. and Dantes, R.,** Patient compliance and the conduct and interpretation of therapeutic trials, *Controlled Clin. Trials*, 8, 12, 1987.

11. **Kaplan E. L. and Meier, P.,** Nonparametric estimation from incomplete observatons, *J. Am. Stat Assoc.*, 53, 447, 1958.

12. **Link, M. P., Goorin, A. M., Miser, A. W. Green, A., Pratt, C., Belasco, J. B., Pritchard, J., Malpas, J. S., Baker, A. R., Kirkpatrick, J. A., Ayala, A. G., Shuster, J. J., Abelson, H. T., Simone, J. V., and Vietti, T. J.,** The effect of adjuvant chemotherapy on relapse-free survival in patients with osteosarcoma of the extremity, *N. Engl. J. Med.*, 314, 1600, 1986.

13. **Meinert, C. L.,** *Clinical Trials: Design, Conduct, and Analysis*, Oxford University Press, New York, 1986.

14. **O'Brien, P. C. and Fleming, T. R.,** A multiple testing procedure for clinical trials, *Biometrics*, 35, 549, 1979.

15. **Peto, R. and Peto, J.,** Asymptotically efficient rank invariant test procedures, *J. R. Stat. Soc. Ser. A*, 135, 185, 1972. (With discussion.)

16. **Peto, R., Pike, M. C., Armitage, P., Breslow, N. E., Cox, D. R., Howard, S. V., Mantel, N., McPherson, K., Peto, J., and Smith, P. G.,** Design and analysis of randomized clinical trials requiring prolonged observation of each patient. I. Introduction and design, *Br. J. Cancer*, 34, 585, 1976.

17. **Peto, R., Pike, M. C., Armitage, P., K., Peto, J.,Breslow, N. E., Cox, D. R., Howard, S. V., Mantel, N., McPherson, K., Peto, J., and Smith, P. G.,** Design and analysis of randomized clinical trials requiring prolonged observation of each patient. II. Analysis and examples, *Br. J. Cancer*, 35, 1, 1977.

18. **Pocock, S. J.,** *Clinical Trials: A Practical Approach*, John Wiley & Sons, New York, 1983.

19. **Shuster, J. J.,** EXACTB and CONF : Exact unconditional procedures for binomial data, *American Statistician,* 42, 234, 1988.
20. **Shuster, J. J. and Boyett, J. M.,** Nonparametric multiple comparison procedures, *J. Am. Stat. Assoc.,* 74, 379, 1979.
21. **Shuster, J. J., Krischer, J. P., and Boyett, J. M.,** Ethical issues in cooperative cancer therapy trials from a statistical viewpoint. I. A general overview, *Am. J. Pediatr. Hematol./Oncol.,* 7, 57, 1985.
22. **Shuster, J. J., Krischer, J. P., and Boyett, J. M.,** Ethical issues in cooperative cancer therapy trials from a statistical viewpoint. II. Specific issues, *Am. J. Pediatr. Hematol./Oncol.,*7, 64, 1985.
23. **Simon, R. and Wittes, R. E.,** Methodologic guidelines for reports of clinical trials, *Cancer Treatment Rep.,* 69, 1, 1985.
24. **Smith, W.,** Randomization and optimal design (with discussion by M. Zelen), *J. Chron. Dis.* 36, 609 1983. (Discussion 613—614; Rejoinder 615.)
25. **Suissa, S. and Shuster, J. J.,** Exact unconditional sample sizes for the 2 ×.2 binomial trial, *J. R. Stat. Assoc.,* 53, 447,1971.
26. **Tsiatis, A. A. and Rosner, G. L.,** Group sequential tests with censored survival data adjusting for covariates, *Biometrika,* 72, 365, 1985.
27. **Zelen, M.,** New design for randomized clinical trials, *N. Engl. J. Med.,* 300,1242, 1978.
28. **Zelen, M.,** Strategy and alternate randomized design in cancer clinical trials, *Cancer Treatment Rep.,* 66, 1095, 1982.
29. **Zelen, M.,** Guidelines for publishing papers on cancer clinical trials: responsibilities of Editors and Authors, *J. Clin. Oncol.,* 1. 154, 1983.

FIGURE 4. Simple randomization for 1200 patients.

```
12211222221111112111211122121211222211121221121 2
>>>>>>>>>>>>>>>>>>>>>>>>>>>>>>>>>>>>>>>>>>>>>>>>>>
21112112211122212221122111211122121211121211 1221
>>>>>>>>>>>>>>>>>>>>>>>>>>>>>>>>>>>>>>>>>>>>>>>>>>
12212112121222111221122122122212221122212122 2112
>>>>>>>>>>>>>>>>>>>>>>>>>>>>>>>>>>>>>>>>>>>>>>>>>>
21111121212111121111222212121222222111112211 2111
>>>>>>>>>>>>>>>>>>>>>>>>>>>>>>>>>>>>>>>>>>>>>>>>>>
11121222212121112221121112212212211212211211 2122
>>>>>>>>>>>>>>>>>>>>>>>>>>>>>>>>>>>>>>>>>>>>>>>>>>
11112111112221221112212221121221122221111122 2122
>>>>>>>>>>>>>>>>>>>>>>>>>>>>>>>>>>>>>>>>>>>>>>>>>>
22221111122122222211111211121111212212212121 2111
>>>>>>>>>>>>>>>>>>>>>>>>>>>>>>>>>>>>>>>>>>>>>>>>>>
22212222112121211122112122112111211222222211 1121
>>>>>>>>>>>>>>>>>>>>>>>>>>>>>>>>>>>>>>>>>>>>>>>>>>
11211212111111121221121212211212222121121222 121
>>>>>>>>>>>>>>>>>>>>>>>>>>>>>>>>>>>>>>>>>>>>>>>>>>
21121212111121112122112121111112212121112211 1122
>>>>>>>>>>>>>>>>>>>>>>>>>>>>>>>>>>>>>>>>>>>>>>>>>>
21221121122121221221211112221111111211122121 1222
>>>>>>>>>>>>>>>>>>>>>>>>>>>>>>>>>>>>>>>>>>>>>>>>>>
21122221212122212111112121111121222211122121 1122
>>>>>>>>>>>>>>>>>>>>>>>>>>>>>>>>>>>>>>>>>>>>>>>>>>
11212111211221111212112122112122211122111211 1211
>>>>>>>>>>>>>>>>>>>>>>>>>>>>>>>>>>>>>>>>>>>>>>>>>>
12211222211222222111122211111212112112221211 211
>>>>>>>>>>>>>>>>>>>>>>>>>>>>>>>>>>>>>>>>>>>>>>>>>>
11112111211122122212111112222121111211121211 1111
>>>>>>>>>>>>>>>>>>>>>>>>>>>>>>>>>>>>>>>>>>>>>>>>>>
11122222111212222212111121211112122221111111 1221
>>>>>>>>>>>>>>>>>>>>>>>>>>>>>>>>>>>>>>>>>>>>>>>>>>
22221221111212111221222112222222221221122112 1122
>>>>>>>>>>>>>>>>>>>>>>>>>>>>>>>>>>>>>>>>>>>>>>>>>>
21211222122112112211222211111221112121212222 222
>>>>>>>>>>>>>>>>>>>>>>>>>>>>>>>>>>>>>>>>>>>>>>>>>>
11121221112122221122222112122222121122111212 1212
>>>>>>>>>>>>>>>>>>>>>>>>>>>>>>>>>>>>>>>>>>>>>>>>>>
22221222212211211222222222221121122211122221 1221
>>>>>>>>>>>>>>>>>>>>>>>>>>>>>>>>>>>>>>>>>>>>>>>>>>
12211222111222111221221111112121112122112222 1111
>>>>>>>>>>>>>>>>>>>>>>>>>>>>>>>>>>>>>>>>>>>>>>>>>>
11121122121122122212222212212211212122111111 2111
>>>>>>>>>>>>>>>>>>>>>>>>>>>>>>>>>>>>>>>>>>>>>>>>>>
21112121112111221222111111212221112122111122 112
>>>>>>>>>>>>>>>>>>>>>>>>>>>>>>>>>>>>>>>>>>>>>>>>>>
21121121111222111122222112111211222222111212 2222
>>>>>>>>>>>>>>>>>>>>>>>>>>>>>>>>>>>>>>>>>>>>>>>>>>
```

FIGURE 5. Random length permuted block lengths of four or six patients.

```
221112212121221211212112121122122121121122122112
>>>>>>>>>>>>>>>>>>>>>>>>>>>>>>>>>>>>>>>>>>>>>>>>
211112221221121212112212122112211212211122121211
>>>>>>>>>>>>>>>>>>>>>>>>>>>>>>>>>>>>>>>>>>>>>>>>
221221221112122111221122211121222211211122122211
>>>>>>>>>>>>>>>>>>>>>>>>>>>>>>>>>>>>>>>>>>>>>>>>
212121121222121121112221212211211221112212221211
>>>>>>>>>>>>>>>>>>>>>>>>>>>>>>>>>>>>>>>>>>>>>>>>
112122122122111222112212111212212122112121212211
>>>>>>>>>>>>>>>>>>>>>>>>>>>>>>>>>>>>>>>>>>>>>>>>
121212211221112212122121211221121212212121112221
>>>>>>>>>>>>>>>>>>>>>>>>>>>>>>>>>>>>>>>>>>>>>>>>
211222112212112211112211212222111212121112221221
>>>>>>>>>>>>>>>>>>>>>>>>>>>>>>>>>>>>>>>>>>>>>>>>
221122211122121122111221212122112221112211121122
>>>>>>>>>>>>>>>>>>>>>>>>>>>>>>>>>>>>>>>>>>>>>>>>
122211211212221122122121112221221112122221111112
>>>>>>>>>>>>>>>>>>>>>>>>>>>>>>>>>>>>>>>>>>>>>>>>
222211212211112122211222111221121121221121221221
>>>>>>>>>>>>>>>>>>>>>>>>>>>>>>>>>>>>>>>>>>>>>>>>
121122222111112222211111221121222121122111222211
>>>>>>>>>>>>>>>>>>>>>>>>>>>>>>>>>>>>>>>>>>>>>>>>
121122121212221112121112221212211122112222111122
>>>>>>>>>>>>>>>>>>>>>>>>>>>>>>>>>>>>>>>>>>>>>>>>
212122211111122211212212122121212121212121122112
>>>>>>>>>>>>>>>>>>>>>>>>>>>>>>>>>>>>>>>>>>>>>>>>
122121211122122112221121122211122122211122121111
>>>>>>>>>>>>>>>>>>>>>>>>>>>>>>>>>>>>>>>>>>>>>>>>
122221122121212112121221112122112122121122111222
>>>>>>>>>>>>>>>>>>>>>>>>>>>>>>>>>>>>>>>>>>>>>>>>
222111212211212121121121222212112111222111222112
>>>>>>>>>>>>>>>>>>>>>>>>>>>>>>>>>>>>>>>>>>>>>>>>
211122212122211111222111221122122211222111221211
>>>>>>>>>>>>>>>>>>>>>>>>>>>>>>>>>>>>>>>>>>>>>>>>
221211212112212121121222112211222111221211112122
>>>>>>>>>>>>>>>>>>>>>>>>>>>>>>>>>>>>>>>>>>>>>>>>
111222221121222111112212121211212211221221112222
>>>>>>>>>>>>>>>>>>>>>>>>>>>>>>>>>>>>>>>>>>>>>>>>
11212112111222221112121212121122211211222211212
>>>>>>>>>>>>>>>>>>>>>>>>>>>>>>>>>>>>>>>>>>>>>>>>
211122221121212121121212122112222111111222112212
>>>>>>>>>>>>>>>>>>>>>>>>>>>>>>>>>>>>>>>>>>>>>>>>
221121122112121211212212211122112221211212112122
>>>>>>>>>>>>>>>>>>>>>>>>>>>>>>>>>>>>>>>>>>>>>>>>
211212211211222121211212122121211122121222111122
>>>>>>>>>>>>>>>>>>>>>>>>>>>>>>>>>>>>>>>>>>>>>>>>
211222112111122212212212112121112212221112121212
>>>>>>>>>>>>>>>>>>>>>>>>>>>>>>>>>>>>>>>>>>>>>>>>
222111212111212211222121122121211122212111221122
>>>>>>>>>>>>>>>>>>>>>>>>>>>>>>>>>>>>>>>>>>>>>>>>
```

FIGURE 6. One-sided P-values for normal curves.

IF Z WITHIN : P=	****	IF Z WITHIN : P=	****	IF Z WITHIN : P=	****	IF Z WITHIN : P=	****	IF Z WITHIN : P=
> 3.090: .001	**** ****	3.090 & 2.878: .002	**** ****	2.878 & 2.748: .003	**** ****	2.748 & 2.652: .004	**** ****	2.652 & 2.576: .005
2.576 & 2.512: .006	**** ****	2.512 & 2.457: .007	**** ****	2.457 & 2.409: .008	**** ****	2.409 & 2.366: .009	**** ****	2.366 & 2.326: .010
2.326 & 2.257: .012	**** ****	2.257 & 2.197: .014	**** ****	2.197 & 2.144: .016	**** ****	2.144 & 2.097: .018	**** ****	2.097 & 2.054: .020
2.054 & 2.014: .022	**** ****	2.014 & 1.977: .024	**** ****	1.977 & 1.943: .026	**** ****	1.943 & 1.911: .028	**** ****	1.911 & 1.881: .030
1.881 & 1.852: .032	**** ****	1.852 & 1.825: .034	**** ****	1.825 & 1.799: .036	**** ****	1.799 & 1.774: .038	**** ****	1.774 & 1.751: .040
1.751 & 1.728: .042	**** ****	1.728 & 1.706: .044	**** ****	1.706 & 1.685: .046	**** ****	1.685 & 1.665: .048	**** ****	1.665 & 1.645: .050
1.645 & 1.598: .055	**** ****	1.598 & 1.555: .06	**** ****	1.555 & 1.514: .065	**** ****	1.514 & 1.476: .07	**** ****	1.476 & 1.440: .075
1.440 & 1.405: .08	**** ****	1.405 & 1.372: .085	**** ****	1.372 & 1.341: .09	**** ****	1.341 & 1.311: .095	**** ****	1.311 & 1.282: .100
1.282 & 1.227: .11	**** ****	1.227 & 1.175: .12	**** ****	1.175 & 1.126: .13	**** ****	1.126 & 1.080: .14	**** ****	1.080 & 1.036: .15
1.036 & 0.994: .16	**** ****	0.994 & 0.954: .17	**** ****	0.954 & 0.915: .18	**** ****	0.915 & 0.878: .19	**** ****	0.878 & 0.842: .20
0.842 & 0.806: .21	**** ****	0.806 & 0.772: .22	**** ****	0.772 & 0.739: .23	**** ****	0.739 & 0.706: .24	**** ****	0.706 & 0.674: .25
0.674 & 0.643: .26	**** ****	0.643 & 0.613: .27	**** ****	0.613 & 0.583: .28	**** ****	0.583 & 0.553: .29	**** ****	0.553 & 0.524: .30
0.524 & 0.496: .31	**** ****	0.496 & 0.468: .32	**** ****	0.468 & 0.440: .33	**** ****	0.440 & 0.412: .34	**** ****	0.412 & 0.385: .35
0.385 & 0.358: .36	**** ****	0.358 & 0.332: .37	**** ****	0.332 & 0.305: .38	**** ****	0.305 & 0.279: .39	**** ****	0.279 & 0.253: .40
0.253 & 0.228: .41	**** ****	0.228 & 0.202: .42	**** ****	0.202 & 0.176: .43	**** ****	0.176 & 0.151: .44	**** ****	0.151 & 0.126: .45
0.126 & 0.100: .46	**** ****	0.100 & 0.075: .47	**** ****	0.075 & 0.050: .48	**** ****	0.050 & 0.025: .49	**** ****	0.025 & 0.000: .50
0.000 & - .025: .51	**** ****	- .025 & -0.05: .52	**** ****	-0.05 & - .075: .53	**** ****	- .075 & -0.1: .54	**** ****	-0.1 & - .126: .55
- .126 & - .151: .56	**** ****	- .151 & - .176: .57	**** ****	- .176 & - .202: .58	**** ****	- .202 & - .228: .59	**** ****	- .228 & - .253: .60
- .253 & - .279: .61	**** ****	- .279 & - .305: .62	**** ****	- .305 & - .332: .63	**** ****	- .332 & - .358: .64	**** ****	- .358 & - .385: .65
- .385 & - .412: .66	**** ****	- .412 & -0.44: .67	**** ****	-0.44 & - .468 : .68	**** ****	- .468 & - .496: .69	**** ****	- .496 & - .524: .70
- .524 & - .553: .71	**** ****	- .553 & - .583: .72	**** ****	- .583 & - .613: .73	**** ****	- .613 & - .643: .74	**** ****	- .643 & - .674: .75
- .674 & - .706: .76	**** ****	- .706 & - .739: .77	**** ****	- .739 & - .772: .78	**** ****	- .772 & - .806: .79	**** ****	- .806 & - .842: .80
- .842 & - .878: .81	**** ****	- .878 & - .915: .82	**** ****	- .915 & - .954: .83	**** ****	- .954 & - .994: .84	**** ****	- .994 & -1.04: .85
-1.04 & -1.08: .86	**** ****	-1.08 & -1.13: .87	**** ****	-1.13 & -1.17: .88	**** ****	-1.17 & -1.23: .89	**** ****	-1.23 & -1.28: .90
-1.28 & -1.34: .91	**** ****	-1.34 & -1.41: .92	**** ****	-1.41 & -1.48: .93	**** ****	-1.48 & -1.55: .94	**** ****	-1.55 & -1.64: .95
-1.64 & -1.75: .96	****	-1.75 & -1.88: .97	****	-1.88 & -2.05: .98	****	-2.05 & -2.33: .99	****	-2.33 > : 1

FIGURE 7. Two-sided P-values for normal curves; ignore sign of Z + VS -.

IF Z WITHIN: P=	****	IF Z WITHIN: P=	****	IF Z WITHIN: P=	****	IF Z WITHIN: P=	****	IF Z WITHIN: P=
> 3.291: .001	**** ****	3.291 & 3.090: .002	**** ****	3.090 & 2.968: .003	**** ****	2.968 & 2.878: .004	**** ****	2.878 & 2.807: .005
2.807 & 2.748: .006	**** ****	2.748 & 2.697: .007	**** ****	2.697 & 2.652: .008	**** ****	2.652 & 2.612: .009	**** ****	2.612 & 2.576: .010
2.576 & 2.512: .012	**** ****	2.512 & 2.457: .014	**** ****	2.457 & 2.409: .016	**** ****	2.409 & 2.366: .018	**** ****	2.366 & 2.326: .020
2.326 & 2.290: .022	**** ****	2.290 & 2.257: .024	**** ****	2.257 & 2.226: .026	**** ****	2.226 & 2.197: .028	**** ****	2.197 & 2.170: .030
2.170 & 2.144: .032	**** ****	2.144 & 2.120: .034	**** ****	2.120 & 2.097: .036	**** ****	2.097 & 2.075: .038	**** ****	2.075 & 2.054: .040
2.054 & 2.034: .042	**** ****	2.034 & 2.014: .044	**** ****	2.014 & 1.995: .046	**** ****	1.995 & 1.977: .048	**** ****	1.977 & 1.960: .050
1.960 & 1.919: .055	**** ****	1.919 & 1.881: .060	**** ****	1.881 & 1.845: .065	**** ****	1.845 & 1.812: .070	**** ****	1.812 & 1.780: .075
1.780 & 1.751: .080	**** ****	1.751 & 1.722: .085	**** ****	1.722 & 1.695: .090	**** ****	1.695 & 1.670: .095	**** ****	1.670 & 1.645: .100
1.645 & 1.598: 0.11	**** ****	1.598 & 1.555: 0.12	**** ****	1.555 & 1.514: 0.13	**** ****	1.514 & 1.476: 0.14	**** ****	1.476 & 1.440: 0.15
1.440 & 1.405: 0.16	**** ****	1.405 & 1.372: 0.17	**** ****	1.372 & 1.341: 0.18	**** ****	1.341 & 1.311: 0.19	**** ****	1.311 & 1.282: 0.20
1.282 & 1.254: 0.21	**** ****	1.254 & 1.227: 0.22	**** ****	1.227 & 1.200: 0.23	**** ****	1.200 & 1.175: 0.24	**** ****	1.175 & 1.150: 0.25
1.150 & 1.126: 0.26	**** ****	1.126 & 1.103: 0.27	**** ****	1.103 & 1.080: 0.28	**** ****	1.080 & 1.058: 0.29	**** ****	1.058 & 1.036: 0.30
1.036 & 1.015: 0.31	**** ****	1.015 & 0.994: 0.32	**** ****	0.994 & 0.974: 0.33	**** ****	0.974 & 0.954: 0.34	**** ****	0.954 & 0.935: 0.35
0.935 & 0.915: 0.36	**** ****	0.915 & 0.896: .037	**** ****	0.896 & 0.878: 0.38	**** ****	0.878 & 0.860: 0.39	**** ****	0.860 & 0.842: 0.40
0.842 & 0.824: 0.41	**** ****	0.824 & 0.806: 0.42	**** ****	0.806 & 0.789: 0.43	**** ****	0.789 & 0.772: 0.44	**** ****	0.772 & 0.755: 0.45
0.755 & 0.739: 0.46	**** ****	0.739 & 0.722: 0.47	**** ****	0.772 & 0.706: 0.48	**** ****	0.706 & 0.690: 0.49	**** ****	0.690 & 0.674: 0.50
0.674 & 0.659: 0.51	**** ****	0.659 & 0.643: 0.52	**** ****	0.643 & 0.628: 0.53	**** ****	0.628 & 0.613: 0.54	**** ****	0.613 & 0.598: 0.55
0.598 & 0.583: 0.56	**** ****	0.583 & 0.568: 0.57	**** ****	0.568 & 0.553: 0.58	**** ****	0.553 & 0.539: 0.59	**** ****	0.539 & 0.524: 0.60
0.524 & 0.510: 0.61	**** ****	0.510 & 0.496: 0.62	**** ****	0.496 & 0.482: 0.63	**** ****	0.482 & 0.468: 0.64	**** ****	0.468 & 0.454: 0.65
0.454 & 0.440: 0.66	**** ****	0.440 & 0.426: 0.67	**** ****	0.426 & 0.412: 0.68	**** ****	0.412 & 0.399: 0.69	**** ****	0.399 & 0.385: 0.70
0.385 & 0.372: 0.71	**** ****	0.372 & 0.358: 0.72	**** ****	0.358 & 0.345: 0.73	**** ****	0.345 & 0.332: 0.74	**** ****	0.332 & 0.319: 0.75
0.319 & 0.305: 0.76	**** ****	0.305 & 0.292: 0.77	**** ****	0.292 & 0.279: 0.78	**** ****	0.279 & 0.266: 0.79	**** ****	0.266 & 0.253: 0.80
0.253 & 0.240: 0.81	**** ****	0.240 & 0.228: 0.82	**** ****	0.228 & 0.215: 0.83	**** ****	0.215 & 0.202: 0.84	**** ****	0.202 & 0.189: 0.85
0.189 & 0.176: 0.86	**** ****	0.176 & 0.164: 0.87	**** ****	0.164 & 0.151: 0.88	**** ****	0.151 & 0.138: 0.89	**** ****	0.138 & 0.126: 0.90
0.126 & 0.113: 0.91	**** ****	0.113 & 0.100: 0.92	**** ****	0.100 & 0.088: 0.93	**** ****	0.088 & 0.075: 0.94	**** ****	0.075 & 0.063: 0.95
0.063 & 0.050: 0.96	**** ****	0.050 & 0.038: 0.97	**** ****	0.038 & 0.025: 0.98	**** ****	0.025 & 0.013: 0.99	**** ****	0.013 & 0.000: 1.00

FIGURE 8. Values for W in one-sided confidence intervals for approximately normally distributed estimates.

CONFIDENCE INTERVAL: ABOVE ESTIMATE - W SE (UPPER CI)

CONFIDENCE INTERVAL: BELOW ESTIMATE + W SE (LOWER CI)

W	Confidence (%)
0.84	80
1.282	90
1.645	95
2.33	99

Note: SE = Estimated standard deviation of the estimate, = "Standard Error"

Interpretation: Before the study is conducted, the probability that the true value of the parameter being estimated falls below the estimate + 1.654 standard error is about 95%. Thus, after the study is over, we have 95% confidence in the confidence statement. Note that once the study has been completed, the "game is over" and probability is no longer applicable.

FIGURE 9. Values for W in two-sided confidence intervals for approximately normally distributed estimates.

CONFIDENCE INTERVAL: ESTIMATE - W SE (LOWER LIMIT)

TO ESTIMATE + W SE (UPPER LIMIT)

W	Confidence (%)
1.282	80
1.654	90
1.96	95
2.58	99

Note: SE = Estimated standard deviation of the estimate, = "Standard Error"

Interpretation: Before the study is conducted, the probability that the true value of the parameter being estimated falls between the estimate ± 1.96 standard error is about 95%. Thus, after the study is over, we have 95% confidence in the confidence statement. Note that once the study has been completed, the "game is over" and probability is no longer applicable.

FIGURE 10. Survival in randomized pediatric cancer trial entries are in days with + to indicate survivors.

TREATMENT 1 — CONTROL THERAPY

1	1	2	7	12+	16	21+	43	47+	48
53	74	105	120	120	131	140	155+	172	195
195	209	237	252	256	265	287	309+	348	351
353	361	364	365	371	377	377	391	396	398
398	404	413	413	414	431	436	445	449	456
462	464	495	506	514	523	553	571	571	595
605+	605	617	629	641	650	671	700	766	769
772	795	801	802	804	828	844	870	874	898
908	932	949	964	973	977	984	1004	1028	1035
1047	1048	1062	1068	1084+	1158+	1173+	1195+	1321	1330
1367	1372	1442	1476	1514+	1559	1602	1639	1671	1678
1680	1690	1758	1777	1793	1797	1807+	1824	1861+	1922
1923+	1929	1935+	1946+	1952+	1984+	1987+	1992+	1993+	2019
2028+	2042+	2064+	2082+	2088+	2090	2110+	2122+	2129+	2166
2186+	2236	2245	2247+	2249+	2277+	2293+	2306+	2308+	2352
2353+	2353+	2405+	2436+	2464+	2465+	2491+	2501	2544+	2546
2580+	2605+	2630+	2640+	2667+	2674+	2678+	2684+	2693+	2733
2763+	2764+	2766+	2772+	2843+	2847+	2878+	2897+	2919+	2919
3018+	3037+	3047+	3070+	3074+	3454+				

TREATMENT 2 — TEST THERAPY

2	4	12	14	15	21	28	32	41	44
75	75	83+	98	98	104	104	133	139	206
213	215	223+	234	244	285+	285	290	313	318
319+	322+	349	357	371	372	375	381	390	394
424	436	443+	443	443	444	466+	475	479	514
531+	537	560	564	586	609	623	633	646	648
656	662	669	704	709	716	720	721	723	748
750	753	758	764	772	772	774	779	854+	888
893	912	952	959	959	960	980+	996	1000	1003
1039	1049	1053	1094	1176	1196	1213	1227+	1231	1245
1248+	1255+	1256	1274	1290	1331	1415	1433	1554	1572
1665+	1690	1700	1714+	1727+	1727	1767+	1772+	1779+	1779
1829	1835+	1842	1847	1848	1871+	1880+	1886+	1905+	1912
1914	1922+	1939	1961+	1983+	1987+	1992+	2003	2004+	2009
2029+	2051+	2051+	2058	2063+	2067+	2072+	2079+	2087+	2089
2121+	2145+	2154+	2155+	2174+	2195+	2196+	2213+	2241+	2254
2310+	2329+	2381+	2414+	2418+	2423+	2441	2447+	2453+	2497
2523+	2526+	2545+	2548+	2554+	2560+	2583+	2589+	2605+	2657
2671+	2697+	2714+	2714+	2719+	2723+	2730+	2736+	2744+	2746
2771	2772+	2815+	2841+	2863+	2863+	2876+	2928+	2957+	2959
2972+	3010+	3017+	3139+	3244+	3310+	3337+			

FIGURE 11. Survival comparison. See Figure 10 for raw data.

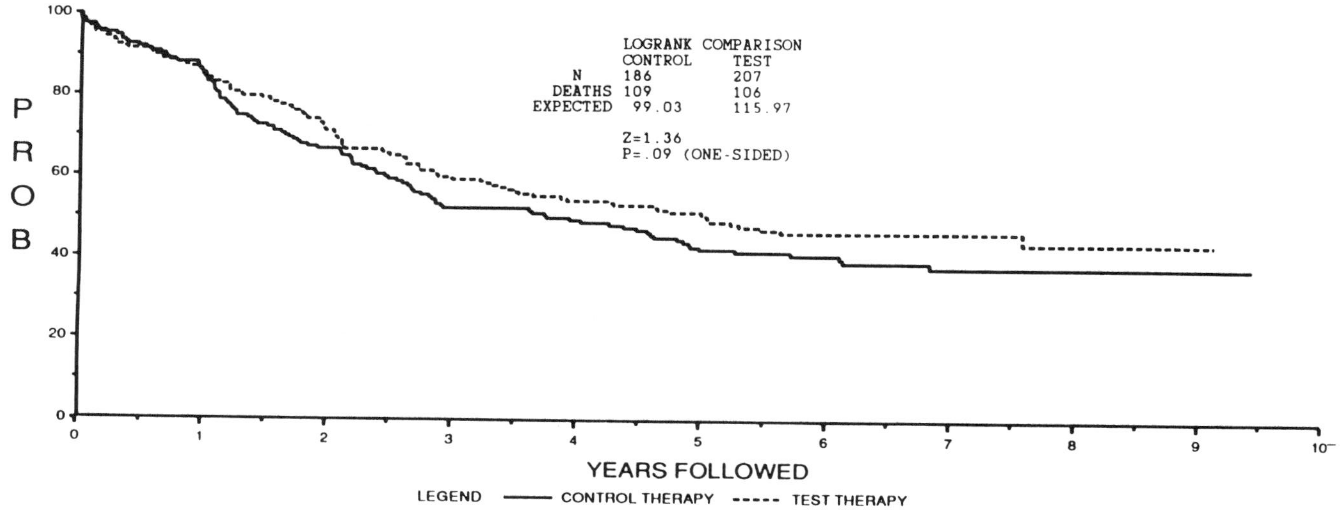

P=EST % FAILURE-FREE THRU END OF INTERVAL
SE=STANDARD ERROR OF P
F=NUMBER OF FAILURES IN INTERVAL
N=NUMBER AT RISK AT START OF INTERVAL

INTERVAL	CONTROL THERAPY P(SE)[F/ N]	TEST THERAPY P(SE)[F/ N]
0– 1 YR	84.6(2.7)[28/ 186]	85.9(2.5)[29/ 207]
1– 2 YR	66.2(3.5)[33/ 152]	70.7(3.3)[30/ 173]
2– 3 YR	51.6(3.8)[26/ 118]	58.9(3.6)[23/ 138]
3– 4 YR	48.7(3.8)[5/ 91]	53.5(3.7)[10/ 113]
4– 5 YR	41.5(3.9)[12/ 83]	50.8(3.8)[5/ 99]
5– 6 YR	40.1(4.6)[2/ 68]	45.8(4.7)[8/ 87]
6– 7 YR	37.0(5.8)[3/ 45]	45.8(6.0)[0/ 52]
7– 8 YR	37.0(12.0)[0/ 26]	43.1(10.3)[1/ 32]
8– 9 YR	37.0(29.4)[0/ 6]	43.1(23.0)[0/ 10]
9–10 YR	. (.)[0/ 1]	. (.)[0/ 2]

Chapter 3

DERIVATION OF THE STATISTICAL RESULTS

In this section, we shall demonstrate the plausibility of the large sample results, while pointing to the gap in the derivation. The mathematical sophistication of a formal proof is well beyond the scope of this Handbook. The aim of this partial derivation is to keep the mathematical level at that of a reader who has completed one year of Mathematical Statistics. More advanced readers are referred to Crowley (1974) and Breslow and Crowley (1974) for complete derivations.

To avoid complicated "stochastic processes", we shall initially make the following artificial assumption. Imagine that for each treatment there is a potentially infinite source of patients. Imagine further that for treatment 1, we shall pick sample sizes of N_1 day #1's, N_2 day #2's, N_3 day #3's, etc. Similarly, for treatment 2, we shall pick sample sizes of M_1 day#1's, M_2 day #2's, M_3 day#3's, etc. For each day, j, we shall restrict our analysis to the first N_j patients on treatment 1 at risk on day j and the first M_j patients on treatment 2 at risk on day j. We assume that the M_j and N_j are selected in advance.

Of course, this not a practical way to conduct a trial. The best we usually can do in practice is to pick N_1 and M_1. The fate of the patient forces the actual values of the remaining N's and M's to be random. Further, since the recruitment process has staggered entry, the actual N's an M's are hard to control. Nonetheless, our artificial method of restricting the analysis allows us to treat the sample sizes (N's and M's) as fixed, and the outcomes on each treatment by day combination as independent binomial variables. The gap in applying the large sample results, as if the actual day-specific sample sizes were in fact planned, can be closed by more advanced "stochastic process" methodology. Intuitively, the percent error caused by using the actual sample sizes versus the non-random sample sizes equated to the expected sample sizes is negligible.

In summary, we shall prove our results under this artificial assumption. We shall argue that the results hold in general on the basis of intuition.

The attached notation chart will be useful in the derivations. Further, Appendix I gives a review of mathematical statistics topics used in the derivation of our results.

NOTATION CHART

	TREATMENT 1	TREATMENT 2
1. j	Patient Day #	Patient Day #
2. Patients at Risk at Start of Day j	N_j	M_j
3. Failures on Day j	F_j	G_j
4. Probability of Surviving Day j given alive at start of Day j	P_j	R_j
5. Probability of Failing on Day j given alive at start of Day j	Q_j	T_j
6. Estimate of Parameter in 4	$\hat{P}_j = (N_j\text{-}F_j)/N_j$	$\hat{R}_j = (M_j\text{-}G_j)/M_j$
7. Estimate of Parameter in 5	$\hat{Q}_j = F_j/N_j$	$\hat{T}_j = G_j/M_j$
8. Cumulative Probability of Surviving at Least k days	$S_k = \prod_{j=1}^{k} P_j$	N/A
9. Estimate of S_k (Kaplan-Meier)	$\hat{S}_k = \prod_{j=1}^{k} \hat{P}_j$	N/A
10. D_k (Estimate Error of $\hat{S}_k$)	$D_k^2 = S_k^2 \sum_{j=1}^{k} \left\{Q_j/(P_jN_j)\right\}$	N/A
11. $\hat{D}_k$ (Estimate of D_k)(Greenwood)	$\hat{D}_k^2 = \hat{S}_k^2 \sum_{j=1}^{k} \left\{\hat{Q}_j/(\hat{P}_jN_j)\right\}$	N/A
12. E_j = Expected Failures (Logrank)	$E_j = (F_j + G_j)\left\{N_j/(N_j + M_j)\right\}$	

3.1 Derivation of the Large Sample Distribution of the Logrank Statistic

Consider the following null Hypothesis:

$$H_0 : \text{Treatment 1 has the same survival curve as Treatment 2.}$$

In terms of the parameters in item 4 of the Notation Chart, this is equivalent to

$$H_0 : P_j = R_j \text{ for all j}$$

The "logrank" test is sensitive to

$$H_0 : P_j = R_j \text{ for all j}$$

against

$$H_A^1 : P_j > R_j \text{ for all j} \qquad \text{(Treatment 2 Superior)}$$

or

$$H_A^2 : P_j < R_j \text{ for all j} \qquad \text{(Treatment 1 Superior)}$$

or a two sided alternative

$$H_A^3 : H_A^1 \text{ or } H_A^2.$$

When mixed behavior occurs under H_A, some $P_j < R_j$ while other $P_j > R_j$, the logrank test may not have good performance.

Structurally, we compute the following quantities relevant to Treatment 1:

$$O = \sum_j F_j \qquad \text{(observed failures on Treatment 1),} \tag{1.1}$$

$$X = \sum_j E_j \qquad \text{(expected failures on Treatment 1),} \tag{1.2}$$

where

$$E_j = \frac{(F_j + G_j)N_j}{N_j + M_j} \tag{1.3}$$

and

$$SE^2 = \sum_j \frac{N_j M_j (F_j + G_j)(N_j + M_j - F_j - G_j)}{(N_j + M_j)^2 (N_j + M_j - 1)}. \tag{1.4}$$

If $N_j + M_j = 1$, then the jth term in (1.4) is defined as zero. The logrank statistic is

$$Z = \frac{O - X}{SE} \tag{1.5}$$

which under mild regularity conditions is asymptotically standard normal under H_0.

Note: If we interchange the definition of Treatment 1 and Treatment 2, all we do is change the sign of Z.

The P-value is obtained from (1.5) and Figure 6 or Figure 7, depending on the Alternative Hypothesis.

Large Sample Result (Logrank)

If the assumptions below hold, then Z given in (1.5) is asymptotically standard normal.

Assumptions:

(a) $\sum_j \frac{N_j M_j P_j Q_j}{N_j + M_j} \to \infty.$

(b) No day is a "wipeout." There exists a positive number $\delta < 1$ such that

$P_j > 1 - \delta$ for all j.

This is equivalent to bounding the failure rates away from one,

i.e., $Q_j < \delta$ for all j. $(Q_j = 1 - P_j)$

Plan of the Proof:

Step 1: Representation of Numerator of Z.

Prove $$O - X = \sum_j \frac{(M_j F_j - N_j G_j)}{N_j + M_j} \tag{1.6}$$

with

F_j Binomial with Parameters N_j and Q_j

G_j Binomial with Parameters N_j and T_j

and $\{F_j\}$, $\{G_j\}$ mutually independent.

Step 2:

$$\frac{O - X}{V} \xrightarrow{D} N(0, 1)$$

where

$$V^2 = \sum_j \frac{N_j M_j P_j Q_j}{N_j + M_j}. \tag{1.7}$$

See A93 for a definition of convergence in distribution ($\xrightarrow{D}$).

Step 3: If Y is binomial with parameter Q and sample size N, then for $P = 1 - Q$

$$E\{Y(N-Y)\} = N(N-1)PQ$$

and

$$\mathrm{Var}\{Y(N-Y)\} \le N(N-1)^2 PQ.$$

Step 4: Show

$$\frac{SE^2}{V^2} \xrightarrow{P} 1.$$

Step 5: Complete the proof.

Show that Z, defined in (1.5) converges in distribution to the standard normal.

Proof of Step 1:

$$
\begin{aligned}
O - X &= \sum_j F_j - \sum_j E_j \\
&= \sum_j F_j - \sum_j \frac{(F_j + G_j)N_j}{N_j + M_j} \\
&= \sum_j \left\{ F_j - \frac{(F_j + G_j)N_j}{N_j + M_j} \right\} \\
&= \sum_j \left\{ \frac{(N_j + M_j)F_j - (F_j + G_j)N_j}{N_j + M_j} \right\} \\
&= \sum_j \frac{(M_j F_j - N_j G_j)}{N_j + M_j}.
\end{aligned} \tag{1.8}
$$

Now F_j is Binomial with parameters N_j and Q_j

G_j is Binomial with parameters M_j and T_j

from the model assumed in the introduction to Chapter 3. This completes Step 1.

Proof of Step 2:

Let us represent the F_j and G_j as Bernoulli Random Variables, and apply the central limit theorem for Bernoulli variables.

$$F_j = \sum_{i=1}^{N_j} Y_{ij_1}$$

$$G_j = \sum_{i=1}^{M_j} Y_{ij_2}$$

with $Y_{ij_\ell} = 1$ or 0 depending respectively on whether for treatment ℓ, the ith patient trial on day j results in a failure or survival.

From (1.8),

$$O - X = \sum_j \sum_{i=1}^{N_j} \frac{M_j Y_{ij_1}}{N_j + M_j} - \sum_j \sum_{i=1}^{M_j} \frac{N_j Y_{ij_2}}{N_j + M_j} \tag{1.9}$$

Using (1.9) and the null hypothesis $Q_j = T_j$ we have

$$E(O\text{-}X) = \sum_j \sum_{i=1}^{N_j} \frac{M_j Q_j}{N_j + M_j} - \sum_j \sum_{i=1}^{M_j} \frac{N_j T_j}{N_j + M_j}$$

$$= \sum_j \frac{N_j M_j}{N_j + M_j} (Q_j - T_j) = 0;$$

$$Var(O\text{-}X) = \sum_j \sum_{i=1}^{N_j} \frac{M_j^2}{(N_j + M_j)^2} P_j Q_j + \sum_j \sum_{i=1}^{M_j} \frac{N_j^2}{(N_j + M_j)^2} R_j T_j$$

$$= \sum_j \left\{ \frac{M_j^2 N_j + N_j^2 M_j}{(N_j + M_j)^2} \right\} P_j Q_j \qquad \left(P_j Q_j = R_j T_j\right)$$

$$= \sum_j \frac{N_j M_j}{N_j + M_j} P_j Q_j$$

$$= V^2. \qquad \left(\text{From } (1.7)\right)$$

We wish to apply the Central Limit Theorem for Bernoulli Variables: (Condition 2), See **A107**

Let

$$b_{ijk} = \frac{M_j}{N_j + M_j} \qquad k = 1$$

$$= \frac{-N_j}{N_j + M_j} \qquad k = 2$$

From (1.9)

$$O - X = \sum_j \sum_{i=1}^{N_j} b_{ij1} Y_{ij1} + \sum_j \sum_{i=1}^{M_j} b_{ij2} Y_{ij2}$$

with

$$\sum_j \sum_{i=1}^{N_j} b_{ij1}^2 P_j Q_j + \sum_j \sum_{i=1}^{M_j} b_{ij2}^2 P_j Q_j = V^2.$$

Now $V^2 \to \infty$. (Assumption (a))

To apply condition 2 of **A107** we must show

$$\frac{W}{V^3} \to 0 \text{ where}$$

$$W = \sum_j \sum_{i=1}^{N_j} |b_{ij1}|^3 Q_j + \sum_j \sum_{i=1}^{M_j} |b_{ij2}|^3 Q_j. \tag{1.10}$$

Now $$\sum_j \sum_{i=1}^{N_j} |b_{ij1}|^3 Q_j = \sum_j \frac{N_j M_j^3}{(N_j + M_j)^3} Q_j$$

and $$\sum_j \sum_{i=1}^{N_j} |b_{ij2}|^3 Q_j = \sum_j \frac{M_j N_j^3}{(N_j + M_j)^3} Q_j.$$

Thus

$$W = \sum_j \sum_{i=1}^{N_j} |b_{ij1}|^3 Q_j + \sum_j \sum_{i=1}^{M_j} |b_{ij2}|^3 Q_j = \sum_j \frac{N_j M_j (N_j^2 + M_j^2) Q_j}{(N_j + M_j)^3}.$$

Now since $(N_j + M_j)^2 \geq N_j^2 + M_j^2$

$$W \leq \sum_j \frac{N_j M_j Q_j}{(N_j + M_j)}.$$

From assumption (b), $P_j > 1 - \delta$ with δ fixed. Hence

$$W \leq \frac{1}{1-\delta} \sum_j \frac{N_j M_j Q_j P_j}{(N_j + M_j)} = \frac{V^2}{1 - \delta}$$

That is, since $V^2 \to \infty$

$$\frac{W}{V^3} < \frac{1}{(1-\delta)V} \to 0.$$

(The other condition 2 postulates are clearly satisfied since $Q_j < \delta$ (bounded away from one) and $|b_{ijk}| \leq 1.$)

This completes the proof of step 2.

Proof of Step 3:

Let Y be binomial with sample size N and parameter Q. Let P = 1-Q. For now, let N > 1.

$$E\Big(Y(N-Y)\Big) = \sum_{y=0}^{N} y(N-y)\binom{N}{y}Q^{y}P^{N-y}$$

$$= N(N-1)PQ\sum_{y=1}^{N-1}\binom{N-2}{y-1}Q^{y-1}P^{(N-2)-(y-1)}$$

$$= N(N-1)PQ\sum_{j=0}^{N-2}\binom{N-2}{j}Q^{j}P^{N-2-j}$$

$$= N(N-1)PQ. \tag{1.11}$$

Note: if N=1, formula (1.11) holds since both sides equal zero.

Similarly, if for now N > 2,

$$E\Big(Y(Y-1)(N-Y)\Big) = N(N-1)(N-2)PQ^{2}\sum_{j=0}^{N-3}\binom{N-3}{j}Q^{j}P^{N-3-j}$$

$$= N(N-1)(N-2)PQ^{2}. \tag{1.12}$$

$$E\Big(Y(N-Y)(N-Y-1)\Big) = N(N-1)(N-2)P^{2}Q\sum_{j=0}^{N-3}\binom{N-3}{j}Q^{j}P^{N-3-j}$$

$$= N(N-1)(N-2)P^{2}Q. \tag{1.13}$$

If N = 1 or 2 (1.12) and (1.13) hold since both sides are zero.

If for now N > 3,

$$E\Big(Y(Y-1)(N-Y)(N-Y-1)\Big) = N(N-1)(N-2)(N-3)P^2Q^2\sum_{j=0}^{N-4}\binom{N-4}{j}Q^jP^{N-4-j}$$

$$= N(N-1)(N-2)(N-3)P^2Q^2. \tag{1.14}$$

If N = 1, 2, or 3 (1.14) holds since both sides equal zero.

$$E\Big(Y^2(N-Y)^2\Big) = E\Big\{Y(Y-1)(N-Y)(N-Y-1)\Big\} + E\Big\{Y(Y-1)(N-Y)\Big\}$$

$$+ E\Big\{Y(N-Y)(N-Y-1)\Big\} + E\Big\{Y(N-Y)\Big\}. \tag{1.15}$$

The above is obtained by writing

$$Y^2(N-Y)^2 = Y(N-Y)\Big\{(Y-1)+1\Big\}\Big\{(N-Y-1)+1\Big\}.$$

Substitution of (1.11) - (1.14) into (1.15)

$$E\Big\{Y^2(N-Y)^2\Big\} = N(N-1)(N-2)(N-3)P^2Q^2 + N(N-1)(N-2)\Big\{PQ^2 + Q^2P\Big\} + N(N-1)PQ$$

$$= N(N-1)(N-2)(N-3)P^2Q^2 + N(N-1)(N-2)PQ(P+Q) + N(N-1)PQ$$

$$= N(N-1)(N-2)(N-3)P^2Q^2 + N(N-1)^2PQ. \tag{1.16}$$

$$\Big[E\Big\{Y(N-Y)\Big\}\Big]^2 = N^2(N-1)^2P^2Q^2. \tag{1.17}$$

Hence subtracting (1.17) from (1.16) yields:

$$\text{Var}\left\{Y(N\text{-}Y)\right\} = N(N\text{-}1)\left\{(N\text{-}2)(N\text{-}3) - N(N\text{-}1)\right\}P^2Q^2 + N(N\text{-}1)^2PQ$$

$$\leq N(N\text{-}1)^2PQ. \tag{1.18}$$

This competes the proof of step 3.

Proof of Step 4:

Under the null hypothesis $(F_j + G_j)$ are independent binomials with respective sample sizes $(N_j + M_j)$ and respective parameters Q_j.

From (1.4) and (1.11) successively,

$$\begin{aligned} E(SE^2) &= \sum_j \frac{N_jM_jE\left\{(F_j + G_j)(N_j + M_j - F_j - G_j)\right\}}{(N_j + M_j)^2\,(N_j + M_j - 1)} \\ &= \sum_j \frac{N_jM_j(N_j + M_j)(N_j + M_j - 1)P_jQ_j}{(N_j + M_j)^2(N_j + M_j - 1)} \\ &= \sum_j \frac{N_jM_jP_jQ_j}{N_j + M_j} = V^2. \end{aligned} \tag{1.19}$$

from (1.4) and (1.18) successively,

$$\begin{aligned} \text{Var}(SE^2) &= \sum_j \frac{N_j^2M_j^2\text{Var}\left\{(F_j + G_j)(N_j + M_j - F_j - G_j)\right\}}{(N_j + M_j)^4\,(N_j + M_j - 1)^2} \\ &\leq \sum_j \frac{N_j^2M_j^2(N_j + M_j)(N_j + M_j - 1)^2P_jQ_j}{(N_j + M_j)^4(N_j + M_j - 1)^2} \\ &\leq \sum_j \frac{N_j^2M_j^2}{(N_j + M_j)^3}\,P_jQ_j \end{aligned}$$

Now since $\quad \dfrac{N_jM_j}{(N_j + M_j)^2} \leq .25,$

$$\mathrm{Var}(\mathrm{SE}^2) \leq .25 \sum_j \frac{N_j M_j P_j Q_j}{N_j + M_j} = .25V^2. \tag{1.20}$$

From Chebyshev's Theorem **A51**, (1.19) and (1.20), we have

$$P\left[\left|\frac{\mathrm{SE}^2}{V^2} - 1\right| > \epsilon\right] = P\left[\,|\,\mathrm{SE}^2 - V^2| > \epsilon V^2\right]$$

$$\leq \frac{\mathrm{Var}(\mathrm{SE}^2)}{\epsilon^2 V^4} \leq \frac{1}{4\epsilon^2 V^2} \to 0.$$

$V \to \infty$ by (1.7) and assumption (a).

That is, from the definition of covergence in probability

$$\frac{\mathrm{SE}^2}{V^2} \xrightarrow{P} 1.$$

This complete the proof of step 4.

Proof of Step 5:

From step 2, we have

$$\frac{O - E}{V} \xrightarrow{D} N(0,1).$$

From step 4 and Appendix **A98**,

$$\frac{V}{\mathrm{SE}} \xrightarrow{P} 1.$$

Hence by Slutzky's multiplicative theorem, Appendix **A105**,

$$\frac{O - E}{\mathrm{SE}} = \left(\frac{O - E}{V}\right)\frac{V}{\mathrm{SE}} \xrightarrow{D} N(0,1).$$

This completes the proof.

3.2 Derivation of the Large Sample Distribution of the Kaplan-Meier Statistic

Refer to the Treatment 1 column of the Notation Chart.

Large Sample Results

Assumptions:

(a) The sample size on day j, N_j are non-increasing:

$$N_1 \geq N_2 \geq N_3 \geq \ldots$$

(b) No day is a "wipeout". There exists a positive constant $\delta < 1$ such that P_j, the probability of surviving day j is:

$$P_j \geq 1 - \delta \qquad \text{for all j.}$$

(c) There is a minimum hazard on any given day. There exists a constant $c > 0$ such that

$$Q_j > c \qquad \text{for all j.}$$

Note that c can be small.

(d) $D_k \rightarrow 0$. (See Notation chart item 10)

(e) $N_k D_k \rightarrow \infty$.

Conclusions:

(1) $\dfrac{\hat{S}_k - S_k}{D_k} \xrightarrow{D} N(0,1)$. (Standard Normal)

(2) $\dfrac{\hat{S}_k - S_k}{\hat{D}_k} \xrightarrow{D} N(0,1)$.

Note: The limiting process can involve Q_j (the probability of failure on day j given patient was alive at the start of day j), k (the day number at which survival is evaluated), as well as N_j (the number of patients at risk at the start of day j.)

$\hat{S}_k$ is given in item 9 of the Notation Chart, S_k in item 8, D_k in item 10, and $\hat{D}_k$ in item 11. The arrow represents the limiting distribution (approximate distribution). See Appendix **A93**.

Plan of Proof:

Step 1: Show that

$$\hat{S}_k - S_k = H_k + I_k,$$

where

$$H_k = S_k \sum_{j=1}^{k} (\hat{P}_j - P_j)/P_j,$$

and

$$I_k = S_k \sum_{j=1}^{k} \left(\hat{S}_{j-1} - S_{j-1}\right)\left(\hat{P}_j - P_j\right)/\left(S_{j-1}P_j\right),$$

with

$$\hat{S}_0 = S_0 = 1.$$

Step 2: Show

$$\frac{H_k}{D_k} \xrightarrow{D} N(0, 1). \qquad \text{(Standard Normal)}$$

Step 3: Show

$$\frac{I_k}{D_k} \xrightarrow{P} 0.$$

Step 4: Show

$$\frac{\hat{S}_k - S_k}{D_k} \xrightarrow{D} N(0,1). \qquad \text{(Standard Normal)}$$

Step 5: Show

$$\frac{\hat{D}_k}{D_k} \xrightarrow{P} 1.$$

Step 6: Show

$$\frac{\hat{S}_k - S_k}{\hat{D}_k} \xrightarrow{D} N(0,1). \qquad \text{(Standard Normal)}$$

Before formally conducting the proof, some rationalization might be in order. First, Central Limit Theorems apply to sums. Hence, we would like to write $\left(\hat{S}_k - S_k\right)$ as a sum. The astute reader might ask, "Why not take logs?" This would work if each $\hat{P}_j$ was asymptotically normal. However, most of the applications will have a large N_j and a small Q_j (P_j near one). In these situations, the $\hat{P}_j$ may not be well approximated by normality.

The decomposition in Step 1 is motivated as follows.

Lemma (Product Difference to Summation):

Let

$$A_0 = 1 \qquad \text{and} \qquad A_j = a_1 a_2 \cdots a_j = \prod_{i=1}^{j} a_i,$$

$$B_0 = 1 \qquad \text{and} \qquad B_j = b_1 b_2 \cdots b_j = \prod_{i=1}^{j} b_i$$

with each $b_i \neq 0$. Then

$$A_k - B_k = B_k \sum_{j=1}^{k} \frac{A_{j-1}(a_j - b_j)}{B_j}.$$

Proof: By adding and subtracting common terms,

$$A_k - B_k = (a_1 b_2 \cdots b_k - b_1 b_2 \cdots b_k) + (a_1 a_2 b_3 \cdots b_k - a_1 b_2 \cdots b_k)$$

$$+ (a_1 a_2 a_3 b_4 \cdots b_k - a_1 a_2 b_3 \cdots b_k) + \cdots + (a_1 a_2 \cdots a_k - a_1 a_2 \cdots a_{k-1} b_k)$$

$$= \sum_{j=1}^{k} \left(\frac{A_j B_k}{B_j} - \frac{A_{j-1} B_k}{B_{j-1}} \right).$$

The term
$$b_{j+1}\cdots b_k = \frac{b_1\cdots b_k}{b_1\cdots b_j} = \frac{B_k}{B_j},$$

which produces the above sum.

Now
$$A_j = a_j A_{j-1}$$

and
$$B_{j-1} = \frac{B_j}{b_j}.$$

Substitution in the sum yields
$$A_k - B_k = B_k \sum \frac{A_{j-1}}{B_j}(a_j - b_j).$$

The completes the proof of the Lemma.

Proof of Step 1:

First, we apply the Lemma with

$$a_j = \hat{P}_j \qquad b_j = P_j$$

$$A_j = \hat{S}_j = \prod_{i=1}^{j} \hat{P}_j \qquad B_j = S_j = \prod_{i=1}^{j} P_j.$$

This yields
$$\hat{S}_k - S_k = S_k \sum_{j=1}^{k} \frac{\hat{S}_{j-1}}{S_j}(\hat{P}_j - P_j).$$

But since $S_j = S_{j-1}P_j$, this further reduces to

$$\hat{S}_k - S_k = S_k \sum_{j=1}^{k} \frac{\hat{S}_{j-1}(\hat{P}_j - P_j)}{S_{j-1}P_j}. \tag{2.1}$$

Now since $\hat{S}_{j-1} = S_{j-1} + (\hat{S}_{j-1} - S_{j-1})$, equation (2.1) can be rewritten as

$$\hat{S}_k - S_k = S_k \sum_{j=1}^{k} \frac{(\hat{P}_j - P_j)}{P_j} + S_k \sum_{j=1}^{k} \frac{(\hat{S}_{j-1} - S_{j-1})(\hat{P}_j - P_j)}{S_{j-1} P_j}$$

$$= H_k + I_k. \qquad \text{(See Statement of Step 1).}$$

This complete the proof of Step 1.

Proof of Step 2: To prove normality, we shall apply the Central Limit Theorem for Bernoulli variables, See **A107**. Note that

$$(\hat{P}_j - P_j) = -(\hat{Q}_j - Q_j)$$

where $\hat{Q}_j = 1 - \hat{P}_j$ and $Q_j = 1 - P_j$.

Now

$$H_k = - S_k \sum_{j=1}^{k} \frac{(\hat{Q}_j - Q_j)}{P_j}$$

$$= - S_k \sum_{j=1}^{k} \sum_{i=1}^{N_j} \frac{(Y_{ij} - Q_j)}{(N_j P_j)}, \tag{2.2}$$

where Y_{ij} $i=1 \ldots N_j$, $j = 1 \ldots k$ are independent Bernoulli random variables with

$$P(Y_{ij} = 1) = Q_j$$

$$P(Y_{ij} = 0) = P_j = 1 - Q_j.$$

Let

$$V_k^2 = \mathrm{Var}\Big(\frac{\sqrt{N}\, H_k}{D_k}\Big),$$

where

$$N = N_k D_k.$$

From (2.2),

$$V_k^2 = \sum_{j=1}^{k} \sum_{i=1}^{N_j} b_{ij}^2 P_j Q_j$$

where

$$b_{ij} = - \frac{\sqrt{N} S_k}{N_j P_j D_k}.$$

Hence

$$V_k^2 = \frac{N S_k^2}{D_k^2} \sum_{j=1}^{k} \sum_{i=1}^{N_j} \frac{Q_j}{N_j^2 P_j}$$

$$= \frac{N S_k^2}{D_k^2} \sum_{j=1}^{k} \frac{Q_j}{N_j P_j} = \frac{N D_k^2}{D_k^2}$$

$$= N.$$

Note that under our assumption (e), $N = N_k D_k \to \infty$ and hence $V_k^2 \to \infty$.

We next show that

$|b_{ij}|$ is bounded.

$$|b_{ij}| = \frac{\sqrt{N} S_k}{N_j P_j D_k}$$

$$= \frac{\sqrt{N_k D_k} S_k}{N_j P_j D_k}$$

$$\leq \frac{S_k}{P_j \sqrt{N_k D_k}} \qquad N_k \leq N_j$$

$$\leq \frac{S_k}{(1-\delta)\sqrt{N_k D_k}}. \qquad P_j \geq 1 - \delta \text{ by assumption (b)}$$

Now since $N_k D_k \to \infty$

$$\frac{1}{\sqrt{N_k D_k}} \to 0$$

and hence there exists B $\geq$ 0:

$$\frac{1}{\sqrt{N_k D_k}} < B.$$

Thus,

$$|b_{ij}| < \frac{S_k}{(1-\delta)B} \qquad \text{throughout the limiting process.}$$

Further, the $Q_j = 1 - P_j \leq 1 - \delta < 1$ are bounded away from one. $\left(\text{Assumption (b)}\right)$. To obtain condition 2 of the Central Limit Theorem, (**A107**) we must show

$$\frac{\sum_{j=1}^{k} \sum_{i=1}^{N_j} |b_{ij}|^3 Q_j}{V_k^3} \to 0.$$

Now

$$\sum_{j=1}^{k} \sum_{i=1}^{N_j} \frac{|b_{ij}|^3 Q_j}{V_k^3} = \frac{N^{3/2} S_k^3}{N^{3/2} D_k^3} \sum_{j=1}^{k} \frac{Q_j}{N_j^2 P_j^3} \qquad \left(\text{uses } V_k^2 = N\right)$$

$$\leq \frac{S_k^3}{(1-\delta)^2 N_k D_k^3} \sum_{j=1}^{k} \frac{Q_j}{N_j P_j} \qquad (\text{Since } N_j \geq N_k,\ P_j \geq 1 - \delta)$$

$$\leq \frac{S_k D_k^2}{(1-\delta)^2 N_k D_k^3} = \frac{S_k}{(1-\delta) N_k D_k}$$

$$\to 0. \qquad \left(\text{Since } N_k D_k \to \infty \text{ per assumption (e)}\right)$$

Hence, from Appendix **A107**

$$\frac{\sqrt{N} H_k}{D_k V_k} \xrightarrow{D} N(0,1).$$

However, since $V_k^2 = N$, (as shown above)

$$\sqrt{N}\,\frac{H_k}{D_k V_k} = \frac{H_k}{D_k}$$

and hence

$$\frac{H_k}{D_k} \xrightarrow{D} N(0,1).$$

This completes step 2.

Proof of Step 3: First note that I_k is a linear combination of terms

$$B_j = \left(\hat{S}_{j-1} - S_{j-1}\right)\left(\hat{P}_j - P_j\right). \qquad (2.3)$$

We shall use the independence of $\hat{P}_1, \ldots, \hat{P}_k$ to obtain the means, variances, and covariances of the B's. See A45 and A46.

(a) $E(B_j) = 0$

Proof: $E(B_j) = E\left(\hat{S}_{j-1} - S_{j-1}\right)E\left(\hat{P}_j - P_j\right).$ ($\hat{S}_{j-1}$ and $\hat{P}_j$ are independent)

Since $\hat{P}_j$ is the binomial estimate of P_j, (a) is clear.

(b) $\text{Var}(B_j) = \text{Var}(\hat{S}_{j-1})\text{Var}(\hat{P}_j)$

$$= \left[\prod_{i=1}^{j-1}\left\{P_i^2 + \frac{P_iQ_i}{N_i}\right\} - S_{j-1}^2\right]\frac{P_jQ_j}{N_j}$$

Proof: Note that $E(\hat{S}_{j-1}) = E(\hat{P}_1 \ldots \hat{P}_{j-1}) = E(\hat{P}_1) \cdots E(\hat{P}_{j-1}) = P_1 \cdots P_{j-1} = S_{j-1}.$

$$\text{Var}(B_j) = E(B_j^2) \qquad \left(\text{Since } E(B_j) = 0\right)$$

$$= E\left[\left(\hat{S}_{j-1} - S_{j-1}\right)^2\left(\hat{P}_j - P_j\right)^2\right]$$

$$= E\left[\left(\hat{S}_{j-1} - S_{j-1}\right)^2\right]E\left[\left(\hat{P}_j - P_j\right)^2\right] \qquad \text{(Independence)}$$

$$= \text{Var}\left(\hat{S}_{j-1}\right)\text{Var}\left(\hat{P}_j\right). \tag{2.4}$$

Now $$\text{Var}\left(\hat{S}_{j-1}\right) = E\left(\hat{P}_1^2, \hat{P}_2^2, \ldots, \hat{P}_{j-1}^2\right) - \left\{E\left(\hat{S}_{j-1}\right)\right\}^2$$

$$= E\left(\hat{P}_1^2\right) \cdots E\left(\hat{P}_{j-1}^2\right) - S_{j-1}^2$$

$$= \prod_{i=1}^{j-1} \left\{P_i^2 + \frac{P_i Q_i}{N_i}\right\} - S_{j-1}^2, \tag{2.5}$$

since $$\text{Var}\left(\hat{P}_i\right) = E\left(\hat{P}_i^2\right) - \left[E\left(\hat{P}_i\right)\right]^2$$ implies

$$E\left(\hat{P}_i^2\right) = \left[E\left(\hat{P}_i\right)\right]^2 + \text{Var}\left(\hat{P}_i\right) = P_i^2 + \frac{P_i Q_i}{N_i}.$$

Also $$\text{Var}\left(\hat{P}_j\right) = \frac{P_j Q_j}{N_j}. \tag{2.6}$$

Upon substituting (2.5) and (2.6) in (2.4), the result (b) holds.

(c) $\text{Cov}\,(B_i, B_j) = 0.$ $\qquad i \neq j$

Proof:

Since $E(B_i) = E(B_j) = 0$

$$\text{Cov}(B_i, B_j) = E(B_i B_j).$$

Now if $j < i$,

$$\text{Cov}(B_i, B_j) = E\left[\left(\hat{S}_{i-1} - S_{i-1}\right)\left(\hat{P}_i - P_i\right)\left(\hat{S}_{j-1} - S_{j-1}\right)\left(\hat{P}_j - P_j\right)\right]$$

$$= E\left(\hat{P}_i - P_i\right) E\left[\left(\hat{S}_{i-1} - S_{i-1}\right)\left(\hat{S}_{j-1} - S_{j-1}\right)\left(\hat{P}_j - P_j\right)\right],$$

since $\left(\hat{S}_{i-1} - S_{i-1}\right)\left(\hat{S}_{j-1} - S_{j-1}\right)\left(\hat{P}_j - P_j\right)$ depends only on $\hat{P}_1, \ldots, \hat{P}_{i-1}$ and is therefore independent of $\hat{P}_i$. Now $E\left(\hat{P}_i - P_i\right) = 0$ and hence $\mathrm{Cov}(B_i, B_j) = 0$.

The result follows in a similar fashion if $i < j$.

Next, we shall evaluate the mean and variance of I_k.

$$I_k = S_k \sum_{j=1}^{k} \frac{\left(\hat{S}_{j-1} - S_{j-1}\right)\left(\hat{P}_j - P_j\right)}{S_{j-1}P_j}$$

$$= S_k \sum_{j=2}^{k} \frac{B_j}{S_{j-1}P_j} ,$$

since $\hat{S}_0 = S_0 = 1$ and $B_j = \left(\hat{S}_{j-1} - S_{j-1}\right)\left(\hat{P}_j - P_j\right)$.

Using linear combinations per A45 and the fact that $\mathrm{Cov}\,(B_i, B_j) = 0$

$$E(I_k) = S_k \sum_{j=2}^{k} \frac{E(B_j)}{S_{j-1}P_j} = 0$$

$$\mathrm{Var}(I_k) = S_k^2 \sum_{j=2}^{k} \frac{\mathrm{Var}(B_j)}{S_{j-1}^2 P_j^2}.$$

$$= S_k^2 \sum_{j=2}^{k} \frac{\left[\prod_{i=1}^{j-1} \left\{P_i^2 + \frac{P_i Q_i}{N_i}\right\} - S_{j-1}^2\right]}{S_{j-1}^2} \frac{Q_j}{N_j P_j}.$$

Since

$$S_{j-1} = \prod_{i=1}^{j-1} P_i,$$

$$\mathrm{Var}(I_k) = S_k^2 \sum_{j=2}^{k} \left[\prod_{i=1}^{j-1} \left\{1 + \frac{Q_i}{N_i P_i}\right\} - 1\right] \frac{Q_j}{N_j P_j}. \tag{2.8}$$

Now applying the Lemma on converting products to sums, we see

$$\prod_{i=1}^{j-1}\left\{1+\frac{Q_i}{N_iP_i}\right\}-1=\sum_{i=1}^{j-1}A_{i-1}\frac{Q_i}{N_iP_i} \tag{2.9}$$

where
$$A_0 = 1$$
$$A_i = \prod_{\ell=1}^{i}\left\{1+\frac{Q_\ell}{N_\ell P_\ell}\right\} < A_j \quad i<j$$

$$\mathrm{Var}(I_k) < S_k^2\sum_{j=2}^{k}A_j\left(\sum_{i=1}^{j-1}\frac{Q_i}{N_iP_i}\right)\frac{Q_j}{N_jP_j} \le \frac{A_kD_k^4}{S_k^2}. \tag{2.10}$$

The above follows since $A_j \le A_k$ for $j \le k$ and the definition of D_k^2 in the Notation Chart.

Consider (2.9) with $j = k$.

$$A_k - 1 = \sum_{i=1}^{k} A_{i-1}\frac{Q_i}{N_iP_i}$$

$$< A_k\sum_{i=1}^{k}\frac{Q_i}{N_iP_i} = \frac{A_k}{S_k^2}D_k^2.$$

From assumption (d), $D_k \to 0$ and hence if we are sufficiently far in the limiting process,

$$1 \le A_k \le \frac{S_k^2}{S_k^2 - D_k^2}.$$

Hence from (2.10):

$$\mathrm{Var}(I_k) < \frac{D_k^4}{S_k^2 - D_k^2}. \tag{2.11}$$

By Chebyshev's Theorem, Appendix **A51**, for any small challenge number $\epsilon > 0$,

$$P\left[|I_k| > \epsilon D_k\right] < \frac{\mathrm{Var}(I_k)}{\epsilon^2 D_k^2}$$

$$< \frac{D_k^4}{\epsilon^2 D_k^2\left(S_k^2 - D_k^2\right)} \qquad \text{(by (2.11))}$$

$$< \frac{D_k^2}{\epsilon^2\left(S_k^2 - D_k^2\right)}$$

$$\to 0. \qquad \text{Since } D_k^2 \to 0 \ \left(\text{Assumption (e)}\right)$$

That is,

$$P\left[\left|\frac{I_k}{D_k}\right| > \epsilon\right] \to 0$$

for any arbitrary $\epsilon > 0$. From the definition of convergence in probability (Appendix A92), this completes step 3.

Proof of Step 4: From steps 1, 2, 3

$$\frac{\hat{S}_k - S_k}{D_k} = \frac{H_k + I_k}{D_k} = \frac{H_k}{D_k} + \frac{I_k}{D_k}$$

$$\frac{H_k}{D_k} \xrightarrow{D} N(0,1) \qquad \frac{I_k}{D_k} \xrightarrow{P} 0.$$

By Slutsky's Theorem, Appendix A104, $\frac{\hat{S}_k - S_k}{D_k}$ has some limiting distribution as $\frac{H_k}{D_k}$, that is

$$\frac{\hat{S}_k - S_k}{D_k} \xrightarrow{D} N(0, 1).$$

This completes step 4.

Proof of Step 5: This is similar to Step 3, but considerably more involved. This itself is proved by a series of steps, which we shall call "tasks". The ultimate goal is to show that

$$\frac{\hat{D}_k}{D_k} \xrightarrow{P} 1$$

To avoid working with random variables in the denominator we shall consider

$$\hat{U}_k = \frac{\hat{D}_k^2}{\hat{S}_k} = \hat{S}_k \sum_{j=1}^{k} \left\{\frac{\hat{Q}_j}{(N_j \hat{P}_j)}\right\} \tag{2.12}$$

and

$$U_k = \frac{D_k^2}{S_k} = S_k \sum_{j=1}^{k} \left\{\frac{Q_j}{(N_j P_j)}\right\}.$$

The large picture of Step 5 is to prove that

$$\frac{\hat{U}_k}{U_k} \xrightarrow{P} 1.$$

Tasks are as follows:

Task 5.1: (See Notation Chart)

Let
$$Y_j = \frac{\hat{S}_k \hat{Q}_j}{\hat{P}_j} = \hat{P}_1 \hat{P}_2 \cdots \hat{P}_{j\text{-}1}\, \hat{Q}_j\, \hat{P}_{j+1} \cdots \hat{P}_k. \tag{2.13}$$

Show
$$E(Y_j) = \frac{S_k Q_j}{P_j}$$

and hence

$$E(\hat{U}_k) = U_k. \tag{2.14}$$

Task 5.2: Show that

$$\operatorname{Var}(Y_j) = \frac{S_k^2}{P_j^2}\left[\left\{Q_j^2 + \frac{P_j Q_j}{N_j}\right\} G_j + \frac{P_j Q_j}{N_j}\right] \tag{2.15}$$

where

$$G_j = \left\{ \prod_{\substack{i=1 \\ i \neq j}}^{k} \left(1 + \frac{Q_i}{N_i P_i}\right) \right\} - 1. \tag{2.16}$$

Task 5.3:

Show that

$$G_j \leq \left(1 + G_j\right) \sum_{\substack{i=1 \\ i \neq j}}^{k} \frac{Q_i}{N_i P_i}. \tag{2.17}$$

Task 5.4:

Show that if we are sufficiently far enough in the limiting process, there exists a constant B_0 such that for all $j \leq k$

$$\mathrm{Var}(Y_j) < B_0 D_k^2. \tag{2.18}$$

Task 5.5

Show that if we are sufficiently far enough in the limiting process, there exists a constant B_1 such that

$$\mathrm{Var}(\hat{U}_k) < B_1 D_k^6.$$

Task 5.6

Show $$\frac{\hat{U}_k}{U_k} \xrightarrow{P} 1.$$

Task 5.7

Show $$\frac{\hat{S}_k}{S_k} \xrightarrow{P} 1.$$

Task 5.8

Show $$\frac{\hat{D}_k}{D_k} \xrightarrow{P} 1.$$

Proof of Task 5.1:

From (2.13) and the independence of the members of the product,

$$E(Y_j) = E\left(\hat{P}_1\hat{P}_2\cdots\hat{P}_{j-1}\hat{Q}_j\hat{P}_{j+1}\cdots\hat{P}_k\right)$$

$$= E(\hat{P}_1)E(\hat{P}_2)\cdots E(\hat{P}_{j-1})E(\hat{Q}_j)E(\hat{P}_{j+1})\cdots E(\hat{P}_k)$$

$$= P_1P_2\cdots P_{j-1}Q_jP_{j+1}\cdots P_k$$

$$= \frac{S_kQ_j}{P_j}.$$

$$E(\hat{U}_k) = E(\Sigma Y_j/N_j)$$

$$= \Sigma E(Y_j/N_j)$$

$$= S_k\Sigma\frac{Q_j}{N_jP_j} = U_k.$$

This completes task 5.1.

Proof of Task 5.2:

$$Y_j - E(Y_j) = \hat{Q}_j\prod_{\substack{i=1\\i\neq j}}^{k}\hat{P}_i - Q_j\prod_{\substack{i=1\\i\neq j}}^{k}P_i$$

$$= \hat{Q}_j\left\{\prod_{\substack{i=1\\i\neq j}}^{k}\hat{P}_i - \prod_{\substack{i=1\\i\neq j}}^{k}P_i\right\} + (\hat{Q}_j - Q_j)\prod_{\substack{i=1\\i\neq j}}^{k}P_i$$

$$= \text{Term 1} \qquad\qquad + \text{Term 2}.$$

Note that from independence E(Term 1) = 0, $E\{(\text{Term 1})(\text{Term 2})\} = 0$, and E(Term 2) = 0.

From A45 and A44,

$$\begin{aligned}\text{Var}(Y_j) &= \text{Var(Term 1)} + \text{Var(Term 2)} + 2\,\text{Cov(Term 1, Term 2)} \\ &= \text{E(Term } 1^2) + \text{E(Term } 2^2). \end{aligned} \tag{2.19}$$

By independence and the fact that from A43,

$$\text{Var}(T) = E\Big[\{T - E(T)\}^2\Big] = E(T^2) - \{E(T)\}^2,$$

$$\begin{aligned}\text{E(Term } 1^2) &= \left(Q_j^2 + \frac{P_jQ_j}{N_j}\right)\left\{\prod_{\substack{i=1\\ i\neq j}}^{k}\left(P_i^2 + \frac{P_iQ_i}{N_i}\right) - \prod_{\substack{i=1\\ i\neq j}}^{k} P_i^2\right\} \\ &= \frac{S_k^2}{P_j^2}\left(Q_j^2 + \frac{P_jQ_j}{N_j}\right)\left\{\prod_{\substack{i=1\\ i\neq j}}^{k}\left(1 + \frac{Q_i}{N_iP_i}\right) - 1\right\} \\ &= \frac{S_k^2}{P_j^2}\left(Q_j^2 + \frac{P_jQ_j}{N_j}\right)G_j \qquad \text{(see (2.16))}\end{aligned}$$

$$\begin{aligned}\text{E(Term } 2^2) &= \frac{P_jQ_j}{N_j}\prod_{\substack{i=1\\ i\neq j}}^{k} P_i^2 \\ &= \frac{S_k^2}{P_j^2}\frac{P_jQ_j}{N_j}.\end{aligned}$$

From (2.19).

$$\text{Var}(Y_j) = \frac{S_k^2}{P_j^2}\left\{\left(Q_j^2 + \frac{P_jQ_j}{N_j}\right)G_j + \frac{P_jQ_j}{N_j}\right\}$$

This completes Task 5.2

Proof of Task 5.3:

$$G_j = \prod_{\substack{i=1 \\ i \neq j}}^{k} \left(1 + \frac{Q_i}{N_i P_i}\right) - 1.$$

This is a difference of products, to which we shall apply the product to summation lemma with

$$a_i = 1 + \frac{Q_i}{N_i P_i} \qquad b_i = 1$$

$$A_0 = 1 \qquad A_i = \prod_{\substack{\ell \leq i \\ \ell \neq j}} a_\ell \quad i \neq j \qquad A_j = A_{j-i}$$

$$B_0 = 1 \qquad B_i = b_1 b_2 \cdots b_i = 1.$$

$$G_j = \sum_{\substack{i=1 \\ i \neq j}}^{k} A_{i-1} \frac{Q_i}{N_i P_i}. \tag{2.20}$$

Now since $a_i \geq 1$

$$A_{i-1} \leq \prod_{\substack{i=1 \\ i \neq j}}^{k} a_i = \prod_{\substack{i=1 \\ i \neq j}}^{k} \left\{1 + \frac{Q_i}{N_i P_i}\right\}$$

$$\leq 1 + G_j \qquad \left(\text{see } (2.16)\right).$$

Substituting in (2.20), we have

$$G_j \leq \left(1 + G_j\right) \sum_{\substack{i=1 \\ i \neq j}}^{k} \frac{Q_i}{N_i P_i}.$$

This completes Task 5.3

Proof of Task 5.4:

First note that since $0 \leq \hat{Q}_j \leq 1$

$$E(\hat{Q}_j^2) = Q_j^2 + \frac{P_j Q_j}{N_j} \leq 1. \tag{2.21}$$

Substitution of (2.17) and (2.21) into (2.15) yields

$$\mathrm{Var}(Y_j) \le \frac{S_k^2}{P_j^2}\left[\left(1 + G_j\right)\sum_{\substack{i=1 \\ i\neq j}}^{k} \frac{Q_i}{N_i P_i} + \frac{P_j Q_j}{N_j}\right]. \tag{2.22}$$

Now since $P_j \le 1$, $\frac{P_j Q_j}{N_j} \le \frac{Q_j}{P_j N_j}$.

Substitution into (2.22) yields

$$\mathrm{Var}(Y_j) \le \frac{S_k^2}{P_j^2}\left[\sum_{i=1}^{k} \frac{Q_i}{N_i P_i} + G_j \sum_{\substack{i=1 \\ i\neq j}}^{k} \frac{Q_i}{N_i P_i}\right]$$

$$\le \frac{S_k^2}{P_j^2}\left[\left(1 + G_j\right)\sum_{i=1}^{k} \frac{Q_i}{N_i P_i}\right] \tag{2.23}$$

Returning once again to (2.17), we note

$$G_j \le \left(1 + G_j\right)\sum_{\substack{i=1 \\ i\neq j}}^{k} \frac{Q_i}{N_i P_i}$$

$$\le \left(1 + G_j\right)\sum_{i=1}^{k} \frac{Q_i}{N_i P_i}. \tag{2.24}$$

Now since from assumption (d),

$$D_k^2 = S_k^2 \sum_{i=1}^{k} \frac{Q_i}{N_i P_i} \to 0$$

and hence

$$\sum_{i=1}^{k} \frac{Q_i}{N_i P_i} \to 0. \qquad \left(S_k \text{ is fixed}\right)$$

Hence we can find for any constant ϵ, a critical point along the limiting process such that once we have passed this point,

$$\sum_{i=1}^{k} \frac{Q_i}{N_i P_i} < \epsilon.$$

That is, from (2.24)

$$G_j < (1 + G_j)\epsilon \tag{2.25}$$

Since ϵ is arbitrary, let us select its value as

$$\epsilon = .5. \tag{2.26}$$

This implies

$$G_j < \frac{\epsilon}{1 - \epsilon} = 1, \tag{2.27}$$

as long as we are sufficiently far enough in the limiting process.

Substituting (2.27) into (2.23), we have

$$\mathrm{Var}(Y_j) \le \frac{2S_k^2}{P_j^2} \sum_{i=1}^{k} \frac{Q_i}{N_i P_i}.$$

Finally, from assumption (b), $P_j \ge 1 - \delta > 0$

$$\mathrm{Var}(Y_j) \le \frac{2S_k^2}{(1-\delta)^2} \sum_{i=1}^{k} \frac{Q_i}{N_i P_i} = \frac{2D_k^2}{(1-\delta)^2}.$$

As long as we are sufficiently far enough along the limiting process, we can use

$$\mathrm{Var}(Y_j) \le B_0 D_k^2,$$

where

$$B_0 = \frac{2}{(1-\delta)^2}\ .$$

This bound does not depend on j. This completes Task 5.4.

Proof of Task 5.5:

From (2.12) and (2.13)

$$\hat{U}_k = \sum_{j=1}^{k} Y_j/N_j \,.$$

From Appendix A45,

$$\operatorname{Var}(\hat{U}_k) = \sum_{j=1}^{k} \frac{\operatorname{Var}(Y_j)}{N_j^2} + 2 \sum\sum_{i<j} \frac{\operatorname{Cov}(Y_i, Y_j)}{N_i N_j} \,. \tag{2.28}$$

Now from Appendix A50,

$$\operatorname{Cov}(Y_i, Y_j) \le \sqrt{\operatorname{Var}(Y_i)\operatorname{Var}(Y_j)}. \tag{2.29}$$

Substitution of (2.29) into (2.28) yields

$$\operatorname{Var}(\hat{U}_k) \le \sum_{i=1}^{k} \frac{\operatorname{Var}(Y_j)}{N_j^2} + 2 \sum_{i<j} \frac{\sqrt{\operatorname{Var}(Y_i)\operatorname{Var}(Y_j)}}{N_i N_j}$$

$$\le \left\{ \sum_{j=1}^{k} \frac{\sqrt{\operatorname{Var}(Y_j)}}{N_j} \right\}^2. \tag{2.30}$$

Substitution of (2.18) into (2.30) yields

$$\operatorname{Var}(\hat{U}_k) \le B_0 D_k^2 \left[\sum_{j=1}^{k} \left\{ \frac{1}{N_j} \right\} \right]^2 \tag{2.31}$$

From assumption (c), there exists a constant $c > 0$:

$$Q_j > c$$

That is,

$$\frac{Q_j}{P_j} = \frac{Q_j}{1 - Q_j} > \frac{c}{1 - c},$$

and hence

$$\frac{1-c}{c}\left(\frac{Q_j}{P_j}\right) > 1. \tag{2.32}$$

Substitution into (2.31) yields

$$\mathrm{Var}(\hat{U}_k) \leq \frac{B_0 D_k^2 (1-c)^2}{c^2} \left\{\sum_{j=1}^{k} \frac{Q_i}{N_i P_i}\right\}^2$$

$$< \frac{B_0 D_k^2 (1-c)^2}{c^2} \frac{D_k^4}{S_k^4} \qquad \text{(See Notation Chart-10)}$$

$$< B_1 D_k^6,$$

where

$$B_1 = \frac{B_0 (1-c)^2}{c^2 S_k^4}.$$

This completes Task 5.5.

Proof of Task 5.6:

From (2.14) and Chebyshev's Theorem **A51**,

$$P\left[\left|\frac{\hat{U}_k}{U_k} - 1\right| > \epsilon\right] = P\left[|\hat{U}_k - U_k| > \epsilon U_k\right]$$

$$< \frac{\mathrm{Var}(\hat{U}_k)}{\epsilon^2 U_k^2}$$

$$< \frac{S_k^2 B_1 D_k^6}{\epsilon^2 D_k^4} \qquad \text{(Task 5.5 and Def of } U_k\text{)}$$

$$< \frac{S_k^2 B_1 D_k^2}{\epsilon^2} \to 0. \qquad \left(D_k^2 \to 0 \text{ by assumption (b)}\right)$$

This completes Task 5.6.

Proof of Task 5.7:

From Step 4,

$$\frac{\hat{S}_k - S_k}{D_k} \xrightarrow{D} N(0,1).$$

Since from Assumption (d), the asymptotic standard deviation, $D_k \to 0$, it follows that

$$\hat{S}_k \xrightarrow{P} S_k.$$

This completes Task 5.7.

Proof of Task 5.8:

By definition

$$\hat{D}_k^2 = \hat{S}_k \hat{U}_k \quad \text{and} \quad D_k^2 = S_k U_k.$$

Hence from Tasks 5.6 and 5.7 and Appendix **A101**,

$$\frac{\hat{D}_k^2}{D_k^2} = \left(\frac{\hat{S}_k}{S_k}\right)\left(\frac{\hat{U}_k}{U_k}\right) \xrightarrow{P} 1.$$

Hence from **A98**,

$$\frac{\hat{D}_k}{D_k} \xrightarrow{P} 1.$$

This completes Step 5.

Proof of Step 6:

$$\frac{\hat{S}_k - S_k}{\hat{D}_k} = \frac{\hat{S}_k - S_k}{D_k}\left(\frac{D_k}{\hat{D}_k}\right).$$

Now since $$\frac{\hat{S}_k - S_k}{D_k} \rightarrow N(0,1) \qquad \text{(Step 4)}$$

and $$\frac{D_k}{\hat{D}_k} \xrightarrow{P} 1 \qquad \text{(Step 5 and Appendix A98)}$$

we apply the product version of Slutsky's Theorem (Appendix **A105**) to conclude that

$$\frac{\hat{S}_k - S_k}{\hat{D}_k} \rightarrow N(0,1).$$

This completes the proof. (You thought it would last forever.)

3.2.1 Difference Between Kaplan-Meier Curves

Suppose we have two independent Kaplan-Meier Estimators

Treatment 1:

$$\frac{\hat{S}_k - S_k}{D_k} \xrightarrow{D} N(0,1),$$

$$\frac{\hat{S}_k - S_k}{\hat{D}_k} \xrightarrow{D} N(0,1),$$

$$\frac{\hat{D}_k}{D_k} \xrightarrow{P} 1,$$

$$D_k \xrightarrow{P} 0.$$

Treatment 2:

$$\frac{\hat{S}^*_k - S^*_k}{\hat{D}^*_k} \xrightarrow{D} N(0,1),$$

$$\frac{\hat{S}^*_k - S^*_k}{\hat{D}^*_k} \xrightarrow{D} N(0,1),$$

$$\frac{\hat{D}_k^*}{D_k^*} \xrightarrow{P} 1,$$

$$D_k^* \xrightarrow{P} 0.$$

In addition, assume

$$\frac{D_k}{D_k^*} \rightarrow c. \qquad \text{(a constant)}$$

Then from **A108 and A109**,

$$\frac{\left(\hat{S}_k - \hat{S}_k^*\right) - \left(S_k - S_k^*\right)}{\sqrt{D_k^2 + D_k^{*2}}} \xrightarrow{D} N(0,1) \tag{2.33}$$

and

$$\frac{\left(\hat{S}_k - \hat{S}_k^*\right) - \left(S_k - S_k^*\right)}{\sqrt{\hat{D}_k^2 + \hat{D}_k^{*2}}} \xrightarrow{D} N(0,1). \tag{2.34}$$

3.3 Exponential Survival

In this section, we shall introduce methods for analysis of exponential survival data. Curiously, we discuss these methods despite the practical fact that we would rarely be in a position to assume exponentiality in the analysis of a clinical trial.

We introduce the methods for the following reasons. (1) We shall be able to show that the logrank and exponential comparisons of the treatments have nearly the same power when the data are in fact exponentially distributed; (2) Planning of clinical trials is generally done under "Proportional Hazards Models", which implies that by a single monotonic increasing transformation, the failure distribution of both therapies can be converted to exponential. The logrank test remains the same under monotonic increasing transformations; (3) Derivation of power and sample size for trials can be done in a straight forward manner for exponential survival. Because of (1), these calculations will apply to the logrank as well. Due to (2), the calculations can be extended to proportional hazards models.

This section will cover the following topics:

(A) Introduction to the Exponential Distribution

The key element is that

P_j = Probability of Surviving Day j, given patient is on Treatment 1 and is alive at the start of day j, is the same for all j. That is, P_j does not depend on j.

Similarly R_j the corresponding value for Treatment 2 does not depend on j.

(B) Estimation of the difference in daily failure rates.

$Q - T = (1-P) - (1-R)$

where $P_j \equiv P$ and $R_j \equiv R$.

Because of (A),

$$\hat{Q} = \frac{\text{Total failures on Treatment \#1}}{\text{Total days on Test for Treatment \#1}}$$

Similarly,

$$\hat{T} = \frac{\text{Total failures on Treatment \#2}}{\text{Total days on Test for Treatment \#2}}$$

Next, we shall obtain the large sample distribution properties of $(\hat{Q} - \hat{T})$. Unlike the logrank test, this will be done under the "alternate and null hypotheses." The logrank properties were restricted to the null hypothesis.

(C) Relate the logrank test to the exponential test when exponentiality holds. We shall see that the logrank test will have only slightly less power than the exponential test. The power loss will have no practical impact. (Section 3.4)

(D) Derive the sample size for exponential survival under given "planning parameters." (Sections 3.5, 3.6, and 3.7)

(E) Extend the derivation to "proportional hazard models." (Sections 3.8 and 3.9)

(F) Relate the derivation to the sample sizes. (Section 3.11)

(A) Introduction to the Exponential Distribution

The reader is first referred to the Appendix **A70 - A76**.

Note that if the "hazard rate" for Treatment #1 is λ_1, then under Treatment #1

$$P_j = P\left[\text{Survive day j}|\text{alive at start of day j}\right]$$

$$= \frac{P\left[\text{Survive at least j+1 days}\right]}{P\left[\text{Survive at least j days}\right]}$$

$$= \frac{\exp\left[-\lambda_1(j+1)\right]}{\exp\left[-\lambda_1 j\right]} = e^{-\lambda_1},$$

i.e., P_j does not depend on j.

Similarly, R_j does not depend on j, where R_j is defined in a similar manner to P_j, except for Treatment #2.

(B) Estimates of Failure Rates and Their Asymptotic Properties

If the survival distribution for each treatment is exponential, then a significant simplification of the survival analysis can be achieved. Under exponential survival, each day carries the same risk, regardless of how long the patient has survived.

Let us consider the following (See Notation Chart)

$F = \sum_j F_j$ = Total failures on Treatment #1.

$N = \sum_j N_j$ = Total days on test for Treatment #1.

$G = \sum_j G_j$ = Total failures on Treatment #2.

$M = \sum_j M_j$ = Total days on test for Treatment #2.

$Q = Q_j$ (Same for all j) = Probability of failing on Treatment #1 on any day given alive at start of day.

$T = T_j$ (Same for all j) = Probability of failing on Treatment #2 on any day given alive at start of day.

$$\hat{Q} = F/N = \frac{\text{Total Failures on Treatment \#1}}{\text{Time on test for Treatment \#1}}$$

$$\hat{T} = G/M = \frac{\text{Total failures on Treatment \#2}}{\text{Time on test for Treatment \#2}}$$

Provided that $0<Q<1$ and $0<T<1$ are fixed, $N \to \infty$, $M \to \infty$ with $\frac{NQ(1-Q)}{MT(1-T)} \to c$ then

$$\frac{(\hat{Q} - \hat{T}) - (Q - T)}{\sqrt{\frac{Q(1-Q)}{N} + \frac{T(1-T)}{M}}} \to N(0, 1) \tag{3.1}$$

and

$$\frac{(\hat{Q} - \hat{T}) - (Q - T)}{\sqrt{\frac{\hat{Q}(1-\hat{Q})}{N} + \frac{\hat{T}(1-\hat{T})}{M}}} \to N(0, 1). \tag{3.2}$$

Further, if the probability of failure on any day is small, but NQ and MT are large,

$$\frac{(\hat{Q} - \hat{T}) - (Q - T)}{\sqrt{\frac{Q}{N} + \frac{T}{M}}} \text{ is approximately } N(0,1)$$

and

$$\frac{(\hat{Q} - \hat{T}) - (Q - T)}{\sqrt{\frac{\hat{Q}}{N} + \frac{\hat{T}}{M}}} \text{ is approximately } N(0, 1).$$

Proof of (3.1) and (3.2):

We shall prove normality of $\hat{Q}$ and $\hat{T}$ and apply **APPENDIX A108 and A109.**

We shall appeal to the Central Limit Theorem for Bernoulli random variables using subscripts

i = trial number

j = day number

k = treatment number

Y_{ijk} = 1 or 0 depending upon whether the ith trial on treatment k - day j results in a failure or not.

$$N\hat{Q} = \sum_j \sum_{i=1}^{N_j} Y_{ij1} \tag{3.3}$$

$$M\hat{T} = \sum_j \sum_{i=1}^{M_j} Y_{ij2} \tag{3.4}$$

with $N = \Sigma N_j$ and $M = \Sigma M_j$.

To prove normality of $\hat{Q}$, we apply A107-1. If we let $b_{ij} = 1$ in (3.3), and note that

$$E(Y_{ij1}) = Q.$$

$$Var(N\hat{Q}) = \sum_j \sum_{i=1}^{N_j} Q(1\text{-}Q)$$

$$= NQ(1\text{-}Q).$$

and

$$\sum_j \sum_{i=1}^{N_j} b_{ij}^3 = \sum_j \sum_{i=1}^{N_j} 1 = N.$$

$$\frac{\Sigma b_{ij}^3}{\left[Var(N\hat{Q})\right]^{3/2}} = \frac{\left[Q(1\text{-}Q)\right]^{-\frac{3}{2}}}{\sqrt{N}} \rightarrow 0.$$

This yields all conditions of A107-1, that is

$$\frac{N\hat{Q} - NQ}{\sqrt{NQ(1-Q)}} = \sqrt{N}\,\frac{(\hat{Q} - Q)}{\sqrt{Q(1-Q)}} \xrightarrow{D} N(0,1). \tag{3.5}$$

Similarly,

$$\sqrt{M}\,\frac{(\hat{T} - T)}{\sqrt{T(1-T)}} \xrightarrow{D} N(0,1). \tag{3.6}$$

We apply Appendix **A108** directly to obtain (3.1).

To prove (3.2), note that (3.5) implies

$$\hat{Q} \xrightarrow{P} Q$$

and hence by **A98**

$$\sqrt{\hat{Q}(1-\hat{Q})} \xrightarrow{P} \sqrt{Q(1-Q)}.$$

By **A95**,

$$\frac{\sqrt{\hat{Q}(1-\hat{Q})}}{\sqrt{Q(1-Q)}} \xrightarrow{P} 1 .$$

That is,

$$\frac{\sqrt{\left\{\hat{Q}(1-\hat{Q})/N\right\}}}{\sqrt{\left\{Q(1-Q)/N\right\}}} \xrightarrow{P} 1 .$$

Similarly

$$\frac{\sqrt{\left\{\hat{T}(1-\hat{T})/M\right\}}}{\sqrt{\left\{T(1-T)/M\right\}}} \xrightarrow{P} 1 .$$

The conditions for A109 have been established and from A109, (3.2) follows.

This proves the major results.

The final findings are obtained by replacing 1 - Q, 1 - T, 1 - $\hat{Q}$, and 1 - $\hat{T}$ by one, in the standard error terms.

As is illustrated in the example below, the percentage error in doing so is extremely small.

Suppose that the one year survival rates are 50% on treatment 1 and 75% on treatment 2. That is,

$$(1\text{-}Q)^{365} = .50 \quad \text{and} \quad (1\text{-}T)^{365} = .75.$$

Hence $$Q = .0019 \quad \text{and} \quad T = .00079.$$

$$\frac{Q}{N}(1\text{-}Q) = \frac{Q}{N}(.9981).$$

$$\frac{T}{M}(1\text{-}T) = \frac{T}{M}(.99921).$$

$$\frac{Q}{N} + \frac{T}{M} > \frac{Q(1\text{-}Q)}{N} + \frac{T(1\text{-}T)}{M}.$$

Thus, the simplified standard error $\sqrt{\frac{Q}{N} + \frac{T}{M}}$ overestimates $\sqrt{\frac{Q(1\text{-}Q)}{N} + \frac{T(1\text{-}T)}{M}}$.

Also,

$$.9981\left(\frac{Q}{N} + \frac{T}{M}\right) < \frac{Q(1\text{-}Q)}{N} + \frac{T(1\text{-}T)}{M}$$

and hence

$$\sqrt{.9981}\sqrt{\frac{Q}{N} + \frac{T}{M}} < \sqrt{\frac{Q(1\text{-}Q)}{N} + \frac{T(1\text{-}T)}{M}}.$$

That is, the percentage error is less than

$$100\left(1 - \sqrt{.9981}\right)\% = 0.095\%$$

In general, by the above argument, the percent error is less than

$$B = 100\left\{1 - \sqrt{1 - \text{MAX}(Q, T)}\right\}.$$

The following chart illustrates the bound on the percent error:

CHART
Bound on Error by Removing (1-Q) and (1-T) terms from Standard Error of $(\hat{Q} - \hat{T})$

Inferior one year Survival	Bound on Error of Standard Normal Statistic
1%	0.63%
2%	0.54%
5%	0.41%
10%	0.31%
25%	0.19%
50%	0.095%
75%	0.039%

Each entry is less than 1%.

3.4 Application of the Logrank Test When Survival is Exponential

If we knew that survival was indeed exponential we would compare the survival by the exponential test, rather than the logrank test. In practice, we can never be certain that survival is exponential.

A key question is how much better is the exponential test than the logrank test when we do have exponential data. It will turn out that the logrank test does almost as well as the exponential test. The margin of superiority of the exponential test is so slight, that the logrank test should be preferred even when the exponential assumption seems reasonable. The reason is that power loss is minimal, while the logrank analysis gives a valid comparison, irrespective of the underlying survival curve.

First, we shall study the numerator of the logrank Statistic: (See Notation Chart)

$$O - X = \sum_j F_j - \sum_j E_j$$

$$= \sum_j \left(M_j F_j - N_j G_j\right) / \left(N_j + M_j\right) \qquad \left(\text{See (1.6)}\right)$$

$$= \sum_j M_j N_j \left(\hat{Q}_j - \hat{T}_j\right) / \left(N_j + M_j\right), \tag{4.1}$$

where $\hat{Q}_j = F_j / N_j$ and $\hat{T}_j = G_j / M_j$.

Let
$$U_j = M_j N_j / \left(N_j + M_j\right) \tag{4.2}$$

and
$$W_j = U_j / \sum_i U_i. \tag{4.3}$$

That is,
$$U_j = \left(\sum_i U_i\right) W_j.$$

$$O - X = \left[\sum U_i\right] \sum_j W_j \left(\hat{Q}_j - \hat{T}_j\right).$$

$$\text{Var}(O\text{-}X) = \left[\sum U_i\right]^2 \sum_j W_j^2 \left\{ \frac{Q_j(1-Q_j)}{N_j} + \frac{T_j(1-T_j)}{M_j} \right\}.$$

The logrank statistic can therefore be rewritten as

$$Z = \frac{\sum W_j \left(\hat{Q}_j - \hat{T}_j\right)}{\sqrt{\hat{V}\text{ar}(O\text{-}X) / \left[\sum U_i\right]^2}}. \tag{4.4}$$

The denominator is simply a standard error, and hence the key is the numerator in determining precision. (The null hypothesis is used to estimate the variance in the denominator.)

Note the numerator is a weighted average: (to estimate Q - T)

$$\text{Num} = \sum_j W_j \left(\hat{Q}_j - \hat{T}_j\right) = \sum_j W_j \hat{Q}_j - \sum_j W_j \hat{T}_j.$$

From (4.3) the weights, W_j, sum to unity.

The optimal exponential estimator would employ

$$\hat{Q} - \hat{T} = \sum_j \frac{N_j\hat{Q}_j}{N} - \sum_j \frac{M_j\hat{T}_j)}{M},$$

(minimizing the variance of $\hat{Q} - \hat{T}$).

Let us consider

$$W_j^* = \frac{N_j}{N} \text{ with } N = \Sigma N_j. \tag{4.5}$$

$$\text{Var}(\sum_j W_j\hat{Q}_j) = \text{Var}\Big(\sum_j\Big\{W_j^* + \Big(W_j - W_j^*\Big)\Big\}\hat{Q}_j$$

$$= \sum_j W_j^{*2}\text{Var}(\hat{Q}_j) + 2\sum_j W_j^*(W_j - W_j^*)\ \text{Var}(\hat{Q}_j)$$
$$+ \sum_j (W_j - W_j^*)^2\text{Var}(\hat{Q}_j)$$

$$= \sum_j \frac{N_j^2}{N^2}\frac{Q(1\text{-}Q)}{N_j} + 2\sum_j \frac{N_j(W_j - W_j^*)Q(1\text{-}Q)}{NN_j}$$

$$+ \sum_j (W_j - W_j^*)^2\ \frac{Q(1\text{-}Q)}{N_j}$$

$$= \frac{Q(1\text{-}Q)}{N^2}\sum N_j + 2\frac{Q(1\text{-}Q)}{N}\sum(W_j - W_j^*) + Q(1\text{-}Q)\sum\frac{(W_j - W_j^*)^2}{N_j}.$$

Since $\sum N_j = N$, $\sum W_j = \sum W_j^* = 1$, and $N_j = NW_j^*$,

$$\text{Var}\Big(\sum W_j\hat{Q}_j\Big) = \frac{Q(1\text{-}Q)}{N}\left[1 + 0 + \frac{\Sigma\Big(W_j - W_j^*\Big)^2}{W_j^*}\right]$$

$$= \text{Var}(\hat{Q})\Big\{1 + \frac{\Sigma\Big(W_j - W_j^*\Big)^2}{W_j^*}\Big\}. \tag{4.6}$$

Case 1: If $N_j = M_j$ for all j then

$$U_j = \frac{N_j M_j}{N_j + M_j} = \frac{N_j}{2}. \qquad \left(\text{From (4.2)}\right)$$

$$\sum U_i = \frac{\sum N_j}{2} = \frac{N}{2}.$$

$$W_j = \frac{U_j}{\sum U_i} = \frac{N_j/2}{N/2} = \frac{N_j}{N} = W_j^*. \qquad \left(\text{See (4.3) and (4.5)}\right)$$

$$\mathrm{Var}\left(\sum W_j \hat{Q}_j\right) = \mathrm{Var}(\hat{Q}). \qquad \left(\text{See (4.6)}\right)$$

Similarly,

$$\mathrm{Var}\left(\sum W_j \hat{T}_j\right) = \mathrm{Var}(\hat{T}).$$

Case 2: If $N_j = aM_j$ for all j and a constant $a > 0$,

then

$$U_j = \frac{N_j M_j}{N_j + M_j} = \frac{aM_j^2}{aM_j + M_j}.$$

$$= \frac{a}{1+a} M_j = \frac{N_j}{1+a}$$

$$\sum U_j = \frac{\sum N_j}{1+a} = \frac{N}{1+a}.$$

Hence

$$W_j = \frac{U_j}{\sum U_i} = \frac{N_j}{N}.$$

Hence

$$\mathrm{Var}\left(\sum_j W_j \hat{Q}_j\right) = \mathrm{Var}(\hat{Q})$$

and similarly $\mathrm{Var}\left(\sum W_j \hat{T}_j\right) = \mathrm{Var}(\hat{T})$.

This implies full efficiency of the logrank test, in case 2.

In a randomized trial, it turns out that the N_j and M_j stay close enough together so as not to make a practical difference in terms of efficiency.

This is illustrated in the following abbreviated example where Treatment #2 seems to have a decided edge in terms of sample size. See (4.2), (4.3), (4.5), (4.6).

Day	N_j	M_j	U_j	W_j	W_j^*	$(W_j-W_j^*)^2/W_j^*$
1	25	25	12.50	.1694	.1894	.0021
2	20	23	10.70	.1450	.1515	.0003
3	19	23	10.40	.1409	.1439	.0001
4	17	22	9.59	.1299	.1288	.0000+
5	16	22	9.26	.1255	.1212	.0002
6	14	20	8.24	.1116	.1061	.0003
7	11	18	6.82	.0924	.0833	.0010
8	10	17	6.30	.0853	.0756	.0012
Total	132	170	73.81			.0052

$$U_j = \frac{N_j M_j}{N_j + M_j}.$$

$$W_j = \frac{U_j}{\sum U_i}.$$

$$\mathrm{Var}\left(\Sigma W_j \hat{Q}_j\right) = 1.0052 \ \mathrm{Var}(\hat{Q}).$$

Similarly, it can be shown that by switching rolls of Treatments #1 and #2:

$$\mathrm{Var}\left(\Sigma W_j \hat{T}_j\right) = 1.0086 \ \mathrm{Var}(\hat{T}).$$

$$\text{Var}\left[\Sigma W_j(\hat{Q}_j - T_j)\right] = \text{Var}\left[\Sigma W_j\hat{Q}_j\right] + \text{Var}\left[\Sigma W_j\hat{T}_j\right]$$

$$= 1.0052\ \text{Var}(\hat{Q}) + 1.0086\ \text{Var}(\hat{T})$$

$$< 1.0086\left\{\text{Var}(\hat{Q}) + \text{Var}(\hat{T})\right\}$$

$$< 1.0086\ \text{Var}\ (\hat{Q} - \hat{T}).$$

The "relative efficiency" of the logrank test compared to the binomial test, the ratio of variances, is greater than

$$(1.0086)^{-1} = .9915.$$

This implies from A130 that the Exponential Test with 99.15% of the patients in each time frame is less efficient than the logrank test with the actual arrival pattern.

3.5 Exponential Survival with a Poisson Accrual Process

Up to now, we have treated the number at risk at the start of each day as fixed. In this section, we take another look at exponential survival under a Poisson accrual process. The results will be almost identical to the fixed daily sample size, but considerable added insight will be obtained. Initially, consider Treatment #1 only. The notation will be as follows:

Number of calendar days of patient accrual	s
Days from closure to accrual to analysis	t
Total duration of the trial in days	s+t
Expected daily accrual rate (Treatment #1)*	A (For Now)
Daily population failure rate (Treatment #1)	Q
Total time on test (Treatment #1)	N
Total failures on Treatment #1	F
$\hat{Q}$	F/N

Note: s = number of days from the opening of the trial until closure to accrual.

*Later, we shall set the accrual rate at (.5A) for each treatment.

Results for the one sample problem Poisson Arrival, Exponential Survival

(1) $\frac{\sqrt{As}}{B}\left[\frac{F}{N} - Q\right] \xrightarrow{D} N(0, 1)$

where $$B^2 = Q^2\left[1 - \frac{1}{Qs}\left\{e^{-Qt} - e^{-Q(s+t)}\right\}\right]^{-1} \qquad (5.1)$$

(2) $\frac{N}{\sqrt{F}}\left[\frac{F}{N} - Q\right] \xrightarrow{D} N(0, 1)$

Plan of the Proof

Step 1.

First, we shall condition on N(s), the number of patients accrued to time s.

We shall represent, conditional that N(s) = n,

$$\frac{F}{n} - \frac{QN}{n}$$

as a sample mean of independent, identically distributed random variables

$$U_j = V_j - QW_j,$$

where

$$V_j = 1 \text{ if patient j dies during study}$$

and $$= 0 \text{ otherwise,}$$

$$W_j = \text{time on test for patient j}$$

$$= \text{time from arrival to death or closure (earlier of two).}$$

The index j represents a randomly selected patient from the n.

$$F \quad = \Sigma V_j.$$

$$N \quad = \Sigma W_j.$$

$$F - NQ = \Sigma U_j = \Sigma(V_j - QW_j).$$

Step 2: Show that given N(s) = n,

$$E(U_j) = 0.$$
$$\text{Var}(U_j) = 1 - \frac{1}{Qs}\left\{e^{Qt} - e^{-Q(s+t)}\right\} = \sigma^2. \tag{5.2}$$

Step 3: Show that given $N(s) = n \rightarrow \infty$,

$$\frac{\Sigma U_j}{\sqrt{n}} \xrightarrow{D} N(0, \sigma^2)$$

where σ^2 is given in (5.2).

Step 4: Show that conditionally , as $n \rightarrow \infty$

$$\sqrt{n}\left[\frac{F}{N} - Q\right] \xrightarrow{D} N(0, B^2).$$

B^2 is defined in (5.1).

Step 5: Show that as $As \rightarrow \infty$,

$$\frac{n}{As} \xrightarrow{P} 1,$$

and hence conditionally as $n \to \infty$,

$$\sqrt{As}\left[\frac{F}{N} - Q\right] \xrightarrow{D} N(0, B^2).$$

Step 6: Show that

$$\hat{B}^2 = \frac{nF}{N^2}$$

satisfies

$$\frac{\hat{B}^2}{B^2} \xrightarrow{P} 1 \qquad \text{(conditionally as } n \to \infty\text{)},$$

and hence as $n \to \infty$,

$$\frac{N}{\sqrt{F}}\left[\frac{F}{N} - Q\right] \xrightarrow{D} N(0, 1).$$

Note that the conditional distributions and statistics in Steps 5 and 6 do not depend on n, and hence they are valid asymptotic unconditional distributions.

Proof of Step 1:

From our study of the Poisson Process, **A143** we know that given N(s), the number of patients accrued to time s, is equal to n, the arrival times form a random sample from the uniform distribution over the interval from 0 to s.

We need to study the variable

$$\frac{F}{n} - \frac{QN}{n} \tag{5.3}$$

That is,

$$\frac{F - QN}{n}.$$

Now, this can be viewed as the mean of the following independent identically distributed random variables: U_j, $j = 1, 2, \ldots, n$ with

$$U_j = V_j - QW_j.$$

$V_j = 1$ (death on study), 0 (survival) and W_j = time on test.

For each j, independently generate the following two independent random variables:

X_j = Arrival time, uniform on the interval 0 to s

Y_j = Survival, exponential with hazard Q (Mean 1/Q).

Note that since the trial ends at s+t, the time at risk is $(s+t - X_j)$.

If	$Y_j \leq s+t-X_j$, then $V_j = 1$	(patient dies during trial)
and	$W_j = Y_j$	(time on test of patient j is Y_j).
If	$Y_j > s+t - X_j$ then	
	$V_j = 0$	(patient lives to end of trial)
and	$W_j = s+t - X_j$	(time on test of patient j is $s+t - X_j$).

Prior to reading the next body of material, it will be helpful to review Gamma integrals (Appendix A82 and A77).

By independence, and the fact that V_j and W_j are functions of X_j and Y_j, we have

$$E(V_j) = 0\ P(V_j = 0) + 1\ P(V_j = 1)$$

$$= \frac{1}{s}\int_0^s \int_0^{s+t-x} Qe^{-Qy}\,dydx$$

$$= \frac{1}{s}\int_0^s \left[1 - e^{-Q(s+t-x)}\right]dx$$

$$= 1 - \frac{1}{Qs}\left\{e^{-Qt} - e^{-Q(s+t)}\right\}. \tag{5.4}$$

$$E(W_j) = \frac{1}{s}\int_0^s \left[\int_0^{s+t-x} yQe^{-Qy}\,dy + \int_{s+t-x}^{\infty} (s+t-x)Qe^{-Qy}\,dy\right]dx$$

$$= \frac{1}{s}\int_0^s\left[\frac{1}{Q}\left\{1 - e^{-Q(s+t-x)} - Q(s+t-x)e^{-Q(s+t-x)}\right\} + (s+t-x)e^{-Q(s+t-x)}\right]dx$$

$$= \frac{1}{Qs}\int_0^s\left\{1 - e^{-Q(s+t-x)}\right\}dx$$

$$= \frac{1}{Q}\left[1 - \frac{1}{Qs}\left\{e^{-Qt} - e^{-Q(s+t)}\right\}\right] \tag{5.5}$$

For inference purposes, we shall need the second moments.

$$E\left((V_j - QW_j)^2\right) = E(V_j^2) - 2QE\left(V_jW_j\right) + Q^2E\left(W_j^2\right). \tag{5.6}$$

This will be greatly simplified when we show

$$Q^2E\left(W_j^2\right) = 2QE\left(V_jW_j\right). \tag{5.7}$$

$$E\left(V_jW_j\right) = \frac{1}{s}\int_0^s\left[\int_0^{s+t-x} yQe^{-Qy}dy\right]dx$$

$$= \frac{1}{Qs}\int_0^s\left\{1 - e^{-Q(s+t-x)} - Q(s+t-x)e^{-Q(s+t-x)}\right\}dx. \tag{5.8}$$

$$E\left(W_j^2\right) = \frac{1}{s}\int_0^s\left\{\int_0^{s+t-x} y^2Qe^{-Qy}dy + \int_{s+t-x}^{\infty}(s+t-x)^2Qe^{-Qy}dy\right\}dx. \tag{5.9}$$

We study

$$\int_0^{s+t-x} y^2Qe^{-Qy}dy = \frac{2}{Q^2}\int_0^{s+t-x}\frac{Q^3}{2}y^2e^{-Qy}dy$$

$$= \frac{2}{Q^2}\left\{1 - e^{Q(s+t-x)} - (s+t-x)Qe^{-Q(s+t-x)} - \frac{(s+t-x)^2}{2}Q^2e^{-Q(s+t-x)}\right\}.$$

Also,

$$\int_{s+t-x}^{\infty} (s+t-x)^2 Q e^{-Qy}\, dy = (s+t-x)^2 e^{-Q(s+t-x)}.$$

Substituting these into (5.9), the first expression for $E\left(W_j^2\right)$ yields (after cancellation)

$$E\left(W_j^2\right) = \frac{2}{Q^2 s}\int_0^s \left\{1 - e^{-Q(s+t-x)} - (s+t-x)Qe^{-Q(s+t-x)}\right\} dx$$

$$= \frac{2}{Q}\, E\left(V_j W_j\right), \qquad \text{by (5.8).}$$

Hence,

$$E\left(\left(V_j - Q_j W_j\right)^2\right) = E\left(V_j^2\right) - 2QE\left(V_j W_j\right) + Q^2 E\left(W_j^2\right)$$

$$= E\left(V_j^2\right) - 2QE\left(V_j W_j\right) + \frac{2Q^2 E\left(V_j W_j\right)}{Q}$$

$$= E\left(V_j^2\right).$$

However, V_j takes on only values of 0 or 1. Hence $V_j^2 = V_j$.

That is, from (5.6) and (5.4)

$$E\left(\left(V_j - Q_j W_j\right)^2\right) = E\left(V_j\right) = 1 - \frac{1}{Qs}\left\{e^{Qt} - e^{-Q(s+t)}\right\}.$$

Summary for Step 2.

We have shown the following properties of the V_j and W_j given the number of arrivals in the time interval from 0 to s

$$E(V_j) = QE(W_j) = 1 - \frac{1}{Qs}\left\{e^{Qt} - e^{-Q(s+t)}\right\}. \tag{5.10}$$

$$E\left(\left\{V_j - QW_j\right\}^2\right) = 1 - \frac{1}{Qs}\left\{e^{Qt} - e^{-Q(s+t)}\right\}. \tag{5.11}$$

Hence $U_j = V_j - QW_j$ satisfies

$$E(U_j) = 0,$$

$$\mathrm{Var}(U_j) = 1 - \frac{1}{Qs}\left\{e^{Qt} - e^{-Q(s+t)}\right\} = \sigma^2.$$

This completes Step 2.

Proof of Step 3.

Suppose that the number of arrivals, n, is sufficiently large to apply the central limit theorem on the V_j's:

$$\sqrt{n}\,\frac{\Sigma\left\{U_j - E(U_j)\right\}}{n}$$

$$= \frac{\Sigma U_j}{\sqrt{n}} \qquad \text{(From Step 2)}$$

$$\xrightarrow{D} N(0, \sigma^2). \qquad \text{(Central Limit Theorem \textbf{A106} and Step 2).}$$

This completes Step 3.

Proof of Step 4.

$$\sqrt{n}\left[\frac{F}{N} - Q\right] = \sqrt{n}\left\{\frac{\sum_{j=1}^{n} V_j/n}{\sum_{j=1}^{n} W_j/n} - Q\right\}$$

$$= \frac{1}{\Sigma(W_j/n)}\left\{\Sigma U_j/\sqrt{n}\right\}$$

$$= \frac{1}{E(W_j)}\left\{\sum_j U_j/\sqrt{n}\right\} + \left[\frac{1}{\Sigma W_j/n} - \frac{1}{E(W_j)}\right]\sum_j U_j/\sqrt{n}. \tag{5.12}$$

By the Central Limit Theorem, **A106**,

$$\sqrt{n}\left\{\Sigma\frac{W_j}{n} - E(W_j)\right\} \xrightarrow{D} N\left(0, \operatorname{Var}(W_j)\right)$$

and hence

$$\Sigma\frac{W_j}{n} - E(W_j) \xrightarrow{P} 0.$$

$\sqrt{n}\left[\frac{F}{N} - Q\right]$ is the sum of two components: (See (5.12))

a. $$\frac{1}{E(W_j)}\left\{\sum_j U_j/\sqrt{n}\right\} \xrightarrow{D} N\left(0, \frac{\sigma^2}{\left[E(W_j)\right]^2}\right)$$

and

b. $$\left[\frac{1}{\left[\Sigma W_j/n\right]} - \frac{1}{E(W_j)}\right]\sum_j U_j/\sqrt{n} \xrightarrow{P} 0.$$

Hence, by Slutzky's Theorem **A104**,

$$\sqrt{n}\left[\frac{F}{N} - Q\right] \xrightarrow{D} N\left(0, \frac{\sigma^2}{\left[E(W_j)\right]^2}\right) \tag{5.13}$$

By (5.10),

$$QE(W_j) = 1 - \frac{1}{Qs}\left\{e^{-Qt} - e^{-Q(s+t)}\right\}$$

$$= \sigma^2, \qquad \text{(See (5.2))}$$

and hence

$$E(W_j) = \frac{\sigma^2}{Q}. \tag{5.14}$$

Substitution (5.14) into (5.13) yields

$$\sqrt{n}\left[\frac{F}{N} - Q\right] \xrightarrow{D} N\left(0, \frac{Q^2}{\sigma^2}\right). \tag{5.15}$$

Since

$$\sigma^2 = 1 - \frac{1}{Qs}\left\{e^{Qt} - e^{-Q(s+t)}\right\},$$

we see from (5.1), that

$$B^2 = \frac{Q^2}{\sigma^2}.$$

and hence from (5.15), the proof of Step 4 is complete.

Proof of Step 5.

Since n is Poisson with parameter As, we have from **A62**,

$$E(n) = As \quad \text{and} \quad Var(n) = As.$$

$$P\left[\left|\frac{n}{As} - 1\right| > \epsilon\right] = P\left[|n - As| > \epsilon As\right]$$

$$< \frac{Var(n)}{\epsilon^2 A^2 s^2} \qquad \text{(Chebyshev Theorem A51)}$$

$$< \frac{As}{\epsilon A^2 s^2} = \frac{1}{\epsilon As}$$

$$\rightarrow 0 \qquad \text{as } As \rightarrow \infty.$$

(It does not matter whether A is fixed and $s \rightarrow \infty$, or s is fixed and $A \rightarrow \infty$, or whether simply $As \rightarrow \infty$ on any path.) Thus

$$\frac{n}{As} \xrightarrow{P} 1.$$

Since

$$\sqrt{As}\left[\frac{F}{N} - Q\right] = \left\{\sqrt{n}\left[\frac{F}{N} - Q\right]\right\}\sqrt{\frac{As}{n}},$$

and since

$$\sqrt{\frac{As}{n}} \xrightarrow{P} 1, \qquad \text{(Appendix } \mathbf{A98}\text{)},$$

Slutzky's Multiplicative Theorem, **A105**, and step 4 yield

$$\sqrt{As}\left[\frac{F}{N} - Q\right] \xrightarrow{D} N(0, B^2).$$

This completes Step 5.

Proof of Step 6:

Let

$$\hat{B}^2 = \frac{nF}{N^2}$$

$$= \frac{n}{F}\left(\frac{F}{N}\right)^2 \qquad (5.16)$$

Now since from Step 5:

$$\sqrt{As}\left(\frac{F}{N} - Q\right) \xrightarrow{D} N(0, B^2),$$

as $As \rightarrow \infty$

$$\frac{F}{N} \xrightarrow{P} Q. \qquad (5.17)$$

Now given n,

$$F = \Sigma V_j \qquad \text{(See Definition of } V_j \text{ in Step 1)}$$

is a sum independent identically distributed random variables. From (5.10), (5.1), and (5.2)

$$E(V_j) = 1 - \frac{1}{Qs}\left\{e^{-Qt} - e^{-Q(s+t)}\right\} = \frac{Q^2}{B^2}. \tag{5.18}$$

Since V_j is Bernoulli,

$$\mathrm{Var}(V_j) = E(V_j)\left\{1 - E(V_j)\right\}.$$

Given n is sufficiently large,

$$\sqrt{n}\left\{\frac{F}{n} - E(V_j)\right\} \xrightarrow{D} N\left(0, \mathrm{Var}(V_j)\right),$$

and hence

$$\frac{F}{n} - E(V_j) \xrightarrow{P} 0.$$

That is, from **A95**,

$$\frac{F}{nE(V_j)} \xrightarrow{P} 1.$$

from (5.18),

$$\frac{B^2F}{nQ^2} \xrightarrow{P} 1. \tag{5.19}$$

From Step 4, $F/(NQ) \xrightarrow{P} 1$. Application of **A98 and A101** to (5.17) and (5.19) yields,

$$\frac{nF}{N^2B^2} = \left(\frac{nQ^2}{B^2F}\right)\left(\frac{F}{NQ}\right)^2 \xrightarrow{P} 1. \tag{5.20}$$

Now

$$\frac{N}{\sqrt{F}}\left[\frac{F}{N} - Q\right] = \frac{\sqrt{n}}{B}\left[\frac{F}{N} - Q\right]\left\{\frac{NB}{\sqrt{nF}}\right\}.$$

From Slutzky's Multiplicative Theorem **A105** and (5.20)

$\frac{N}{\sqrt{F}}\left[\frac{F}{N} - Q\right]$ has the same asymptotic distribution as

$$\frac{\sqrt{n}}{B}\left[\frac{F}{N} - Q\right]$$

which is N(0, 1) from Step 4.

This completes the proof.

3.6 Extension to the Two-Sample Problem

Here the accrual rate is A/2 to each treatment, G is the number of failures on Treatment #2, M is the total time on test for Treatment #2. T is the daily failure rate on Treatment #2. We have by the one sample results (halving the accrual rate):

$$\sqrt{(.5A)s}\left[\frac{F}{N} - Q\right] \xrightarrow{D} N(0, B^2)$$

with

$$B^2 = Q^2\left[1 - \frac{1}{Qs}\left\{e^{-Qt} - e^{-Q(s+t)}\right\}\right]^{-1}.$$

$$\sqrt{(.5A)s}\left[\frac{G}{M} - T\right] \xrightarrow{D} N(0, C^2)$$

with

$$C^2 = T^2\left[1 - \frac{1}{Ts}\left\{e^{-Tt} - e^{-T(s+t)}\right\}\right]^{-1}$$

Hence

$$\sqrt{(.5A)s}\left[\left(\frac{F}{N} - \frac{G}{M}\right) - (Q - T)\right] \xrightarrow{D} N(0, B^2 + C^2),$$

Since from A142, each accrual process is independent, and A108 can be applied.

Now from the previous section, Steps 5 and 6

$$\frac{B^2/(.5As)}{F/N^2} \xrightarrow{P} 1$$

and

$$\frac{C^2/(.5As)}{G/M^2} \xrightarrow{P} 1.$$

Hence from the Appendix **A103**,

$$\frac{(B^2 + C^2)/(.5As)}{(F/N^2) + (G/M^2)} \xrightarrow{P} 1.$$

By applying **A109**, the following "Block" holds:

Results for Poisson Entry, Exponential Survival

(1) $$\frac{\sqrt{(.5As)}}{\sqrt{B^2 + C^2}}\left[\frac{F}{N} - \frac{G}{M} - (Q - T)\right] \xrightarrow{D} N(0, 1).$$

(2) $$\left[\frac{F}{N} - \frac{G}{M} - (Q - T)\right] \frac{1}{\sqrt{(F/N^2) + (G/M^2)}} \xrightarrow{D} N(0, 1).$$

(3) $$\frac{(B^2 + C^2)/(.5As)}{\sqrt{(F/N^2) + (G/M^2)}} \xrightarrow{P} 1.$$

A = total accrual rate (A/2 to each treatment).

$$B^2 = Q^2\left[1 - \frac{1}{Qs}\left\{e^{-Qt} - e^{-Q(s+t)}\right\}\right]^{-1}.$$

$$C^2 = T^2\left[1 - \frac{1}{Ts}\left\{e^{-Tt} - e^{-T(s+t)}\right\}\right]^{-1}.$$

s = Accrual period. (Calendar time)

t = Time from end of accrual to analysis.

Q = Population daily failure rate on Treatment #1.

T = Population daily failure rate on Treatment #2.

F = Failures on Treatment #1 (observed).

G = Failures on Treatment #2 (observed).

N = Total time on test for Treatment #1 (total patient days).

M = Total time on test for Treatment #2.

Comparison with the fixed daily sample size version. The asymptotic result of section 3.3 was:

$$\frac{\hat{Q} - \hat{T} - (Q - T)}{\sqrt{\frac{\hat{Q}}{N} + \frac{\hat{T}}{M}}} \xrightarrow{D} N(0, 1). \qquad \text{(Approximately)}$$

Since $\hat{Q} = F/N$ and $\hat{T} = G/M$, this result is identical to (2) above.

<u>Sample size derivation</u> for exponential survival with Poisson Accrual.

Please consult Appendix **A130(1)** and **A135**, as well as template on final conclusions for Poisson entry above. We shall identify each term in **A130**:

$$H_0\text{: } \theta = Q - T = 0. \qquad (\theta_0 = 0)$$

$$H_A\text{: } \theta = Q - T = \theta_1 > 0. \qquad \text{(One-sided)}$$

$$\hat{\theta} = (F/N) - (G/M).$$

$$SE = \sqrt{(F/N^2) + (G/M^2)}.$$

$$S = \sqrt{(B^2 + C^2)/(.5As)}.$$

Hence the necessary sample size for Type I error α and Type II error β (Power 1 - β) satisfies

$$S = \frac{Q - T}{(Z_\alpha + Z_\beta)}.$$

This is solved by bisection. See block below for full definition of terms.

Sample Size Equation for Poisson Accrual and Exponential Survival:

Two sample trial with 50% allocation to each treatment. One-sided Test Calculation. (Replace α by $\alpha/2$ for two-sided test.)

$$\frac{B^2 + C^2}{(.5As)} = \frac{(Q - T)^2}{(Z_\alpha + Z_\beta)^2} \tag{6.1}$$

A = Total accrual rate.

s = Total calendar time of accrual.

t = Time from end of accrual to analysis (minimum follow-up time).

Q = Daily failure rate on Treatment #1 (under H_A).

T = Daily Failure Rate on Treatment #2 (under H_A).

α = Probability of a Type I error (Reject H_0 when true).

Z_α = Upper 100α% point of the standard normal distribution.

β = 1 - Power = Probability of a Type II error (Reject H_A when true).

Z_β = Upper 100β% point of the standard normal

$$B^2 = Q^2\left[1 - \frac{1}{Qs}\left\{e^{-Qt} - e^{-Q(s+t)}\right\}\right]^{-1}. \tag{6.2}$$

$$C^2 = T^2\left[1 - \frac{1}{Ts}\left\{e^{-Tt} - e^{-T(s+t)}\right\}\right]^{-1}. \tag{6.3}$$

See Section 3.10 regarding losses to follow-up.

Sample sizes for exponential survival use FACT = 1.0, in the Program.

3.7 Exponential Survival with "Up-Front" Accrual

In rare instances, it is possible to accrue all patients at day 1 and follow them for t years.

We derive the distributional properties from the Poisson Arrival as follows:

Let the accrual period $s \rightarrow 0$.

Let the accrual rate $A \rightarrow \infty$,

with $As \rightarrow n$ (large).

From this, we shall obtain the analogous one sample and two sample results. Recall that

$$B^2 = Q^2\left[1 - \frac{1}{Qs}\left\{e^{-Qt} - e^{-Q(s+t)}\right\}\right]^{-1}.$$

By L'Hospital's rule, letting the accrual period $s \rightarrow 0$

$$\lim_{s \rightarrow 0} \frac{e^{-Qt} - e^{-Q(s+t)}}{Qs} = \lim_{s \rightarrow 0} \frac{Qe^{-Q(s+t)}}{Q} = e^{-Qt}.$$

Hence

$$B^2 \rightarrow Q^2\left[1 - e^{-Qt}\right]^{-1} \quad \text{as } s \rightarrow 0.$$

This limit is used as the B^2 value in the variance formula.

Results for the One Sample Problem with Exponential Survival and Up Front Accrual:

(1) $\frac{\sqrt{n}}{B}\left[\frac{F}{N} - Q\right] \xrightarrow{D} N(0, 1),$

where Q = Daily failure rate.

n = Number of patients treated.

F = Observed failures.

N = Total time on test.

$B^2 = Q^2\left[1 - e^{-Qt}\right]^{-1}.$

t = Time from accrual to analysis (follow-up time).

(2) $\frac{N}{\sqrt{F}}\left[\frac{F}{N} - Q\right] \xrightarrow{D} N(0, 1).$

(3) $\frac{N/\sqrt{F}}{\sqrt{n}/B} \xrightarrow{P} 1.$

Results for the Two Sample Problem with Exponential Survival and Up Front Entry:

(1) $$\frac{\sqrt{.5n}}{\sqrt{B^2 + C^2}} \left[\frac{F}{N} - \frac{G}{M} - (Q - T)\right] \xrightarrow{D} N(0, 1)$$

(2) $$\left[\frac{F}{N} - \frac{G}{M} - (Q - T)\right] \frac{1}{\sqrt{(F/N^2) + (G/M^2)}} \xrightarrow{D} N(0, 1)$$

(3) $$\frac{(B^2 + C^2)/(.5n)}{\left[(F/N^2) + (G/M^2)\right]} \xrightarrow{P} 1$$

with n = Total patient accrual ($n/2$ to each treatment).

$B^2 = Q^2\left[1 - e^{-Qt}\right]^{-1}$

$C^2 = T^2\left[1 - e^{-Tt}\right]^{-1}$.

t = Time from start of study to analysis (follow-up time)

Q = Population failure rate on Treatment #1.

T = Population Failure rate on Treatment #2.

Sample Size Equation for Up Front Accrual and Exponential Survival: Two sample trial with 50% allocation to each treatment. One-sided Test Calculation. (Replace α by $\alpha/2$ for two-sided test.)

$$\frac{B^2 + C^2}{.5n} = \frac{(Q - T)^2}{(Z_\alpha + Z_\beta)^2}. \tag{7.1}$$

n = Total number of patients.

t = Time from start of study to analysis (follow-up time).

Q = Daily failure rate (Treatment #1).

T = Daily failure rate (Treatment #2).

α = Probability of a Type I error (Reject H_0 when true).

β = Probability of a Type II error (Reject H_A when true).

Z_α = Upper (100α)% point of the standard normal distribution.

Z_β = Upper (100β)% point of the standard normal distribution.

$$B^2 = Q^2\left[1 - e^{-Qt}\right]^{-1} \tag{7.2}$$

$$C^2 = T^2\left[1 - e^{-Tt}\right]^{-1}. \tag{7.3}$$

See Section 3.10 regarding losses to follow-up

This formula also can be used when patients are entered in any fashion, but followed for a period t, not longer.

The program obtains this under FACT = 0.

3.8 Proportional Hazard Models and the Exponential Distribution

Let $F_j(x)$ be the cumulative distribution of survival for treatment j, j = 1, 2 respectively.

$$F_j(x) = P\left[X_j \le x\right] \qquad \text{(See A20)}$$

The logrank test is defined for testing the null hypothesis

$$H_0: F_1(x) = F_2(x) \qquad \text{for all } x.$$

The alternative is typically for the one-sided case:

$$H_A: F_1(x) \le F_2(x) \qquad \text{for all } x \qquad \text{(Treatment \#1 Superior)}$$

The proportional hazard formulation adds structure to H_A as follows:

$$H_A: \left\{1 - F_2(x)\right\} = \left\{1 - F_1(x)\right\}^{\theta}. \tag{8.1}$$

If the distributions have continuous densities represented by f_1 and f_2 respectively, then (8.1) can be considered as follows

$$F_2(x) = 1 - \left[\int_x^{\infty} f_1(t)dt\right]^{\theta}. \tag{8.2}$$

Differentiating both sides with respect to x yields for $\theta \neq 1$ (Chain rule)

$$F_2'(x) = f_2(x) = \theta f_1(x)\left[\int_x^{\infty} f_1(t)dt\right]^{\theta-1},$$

i.e.

$$f_2(x) = \theta f_1(x)\left\{1 - F_1(x)\right\}^{\theta-1}.$$

$$\frac{f_2(x)}{\left[1 - F_1(x)\right]^{\theta}} = \frac{\theta f_1(x)}{1 - F_1(x)}. \tag{8.3}$$

That is, from (8.1)

$$\frac{f_2(x)}{1 - F_2(x)} = \frac{\theta f_1(x)}{1 - F_1(x)} \tag{8.4}$$

Now if $\theta = 1$, (8.4), still holds.

From Appendix A75 which defines the Hazard Rate, the alternate hypothesis (8.1) states that the hazard rates are proportional. That is, the ratio of hazards is independent of time. If and only if $\theta < 1$, then Treatment #2 has a lower failure rate than Treatment #1.

The following result relates proportional hazards in a rather remarkable way to the exponential.

Theorem 8.1:

Let

$$1 - F_1(x) = \left[1 - G(x)\right]^{\gamma} \tag{8.5}$$

and

$$1 - F_2(x) = \left[1 - G(x)\right]^{\gamma+\theta}, \tag{8.6}$$

where $G(x)$ is a known distribution but γ and θ are unknown.

Let us transform the time scale x by

$$y = -\log\left\{1 - G(x)\right\}. \tag{8.7}$$

In this time scale, let Y_1 and Y_2 represent random variables of survival times on Treatments #1 and #2 respectively.

Then Y_1 and Y_2 are respectively exponential with hazards γ and $(\gamma + \theta)$.

Proof:

From the Appendix A89,

$$Y_1 \text{ has density } \frac{f_1(x)}{(dy/dx)}.$$

Now from (8.7),

$$\frac{dy}{dx} = \frac{G'(x)}{1 - G(x)}.$$

From Appendix A21 and (8.5)

$$f_1(x) = \gamma\left\{1 - G(x)\right\}^{\gamma-1} G'(x).$$

That is, Y_1 has density

$$h_1(y) = \gamma\left\{1 - G(x)\right\}^{\gamma} \qquad 0 < G(x) < 1.$$

But $1 - G(x) = e^{-y}$ $\left(\text{See (8.7)}\right)$ and hence Y_1 has density

$$h_1(y) = \gamma e^{-\gamma y} \qquad y > 0.$$

Similarly, replacing γ by $(\gamma + \theta)$ in the above yields the fact that Y_2 has density

$$h_2(y) = (\gamma + \theta)e^{-(\gamma+\theta)y} \qquad y > 0.$$

This completes the proof.

This transformation converts a proportional hazard problem to an exponential problem.

3.9 Considerations in Planning a Trial Under Proportional Hazards: Putting It All Together

Suppose you wished to plan a trial with the following endpoints:

Annual Accrual:	150 patients per year.
Two Year Survival:	40% Control (Treatment #1).
	50% Experimental (Treatment #2).
Alpha:	.025 (one-sided).
Power:	80%.
Distribution:	Exponential (For Now).

A total of 300 patients are expected to be accrued through the two year endpoint, and hence from the sample size Program (FACT = 1.0), 541 patients (3.6 years of accrual) are required. The trial would require an additional two years of follow-up.

As we have seen in Section 3.4, the power loss in the use of the logrank test as opposed to the exponential test would be of no practical concern.

However, the key issue one faces is non-exponentiality.

In answering this question, let us first consider an alternate study where the accrual is up front (or similarly if we only use the first two years of patient data.) Suppose further that you were willing to assume proportional hazards. Then the power loss caused by lack of knowledge of G would be minimal, since

(a) There exists a monotonic transformation to convert the data to exponential.

(b) The logrank test is invariant under monotonic transformations.

(c) From Theorem 8.1 the exponential parameters do not involve G.

(d) The logrank and exponential tests have virtually the same power, when exponentiality holds.

* The distribution G plays no role in planning this alternate study under proportional hazards and the planning endpoints.

In the actual setting of follow-up to the end of the study, the key sample size planning issue is what happens to patients after surviving to the endpoint of the study.

In the above example, the study is planned for 3.6 years of accrual plus 2 years of follow-up for a total of 5.6 years. Patients are at risk from 2.0 to 5.6 years.

To accommodate this in a quantitative way, we shall consider attaching exponential survival past the endpoint, but with a lower hazard. Proportional hazards are still assumed. More sophisticated assumptions would result in contingencies too numerous to program.

The derivations will be conducted as follows:

	Daily Hazard Before t	Daily Hazard After t ($d \geq 0$)
Treatment #1	Q	dQ
Treatment #2	T	dT

Non-Exponentiality before the endpoint t will have virtually no impact on the power.

> NOTE: If d=0, no failures will occur after t, and we can use up front accrual results for design and analysis.

If $d > 0$, then the following transformation produces exponentiality under both treatments, with respective hazards Q and T. (Y is transformed time, X is original time.)

$$Y = X \qquad \text{if } X \leq t$$

$$= t + d(X-t) \qquad \text{if } X > t,$$

since for $x > t$, and treatment 1

$$P[X > x] = P[X > t]P[X > x|X > t]$$

$$= e^{-Qt} e^{-dQ(x-t)}$$

$$= e^{-Q[t+d(x-t)]}$$

Setting $Y = t + d(X-t)$ and $y = t+d(x-t)$ yields exponentiality with hazard Q for $Y > t$.

Since it was assumed for $Y \leq t$, exponentiality holds for Y.

Based on exponential considerations, we would estimate Q by

$$\hat{Q} = \frac{\text{Total Failures}}{\text{Total accumulated time on test in Y-scale}}$$

Following the same derivation as seen in Section 3.5, "Exponential Survival with a Poisson Accrual

Process," the following results are obtained:

Let

F_1 = Number of failures occurring prior to patient time on test t.

N_1 = total accumulated time on test accrued by patients prior to t. (Clock only is on while patient is at risk less than t.)

F_2 = Number of failures occurring after patient time on test t.

N_2 = total accumulated time on test accrued by patients after t. (Clock starts for patient after t.)

with other notation per page 96.

Let

$$\hat{Q} = \frac{F_1 + F_2}{N_1 + dN_2}$$

be the exponential estimate of Q on the basis of the transformation to exponential. Then

$$\frac{\hat{Q} - Q}{V} \xrightarrow{D} N(0, 1), \tag{9.1}$$

where

$$V^2 = \frac{Q^2}{As}\left[1 - \frac{e^{-Qt}}{dQs}\left\{1 - e^{-dQs}\right\}\right]^{-1}. \tag{9.2}$$

Before proving this result, note that

(a) If d = 1, we obtain the result for exponentials (5.1).

(b) If d → 0, by L'Hospital's rule

$$V^2 \rightarrow \frac{Q^2}{As}\left[1 - e^{-Qt}\right], \tag{9.3}$$

which agrees with the Up Front Accrual results in Section 3.7.

Proof: Although the proof can be derived exactly as in the exponential case, once $E(U_j)$ and $Var(U_j)$ are obtained, we shall outline an alternate proof.

Step 1: Show

$$\hat{Q} = \frac{F_1}{N_1} W_1 + \frac{F_2}{dN_2} W_2$$

where

$$W_1 = \frac{N_1}{N_1 + dN_2}$$

and

$$W_2 = \frac{dN_2}{N_1 + dN_2} = 1 - W_1.$$

Step 2: Apply results for Up Front Accrual to show

$$\frac{\left(\frac{F_1}{N_1} - Q\right)}{V_1} \xrightarrow{D} N(0, 1),$$

where

$$V_1^2 = \frac{Q^2}{As(1 - e^{-Qt})}$$

$$= \frac{Q}{E(N_1)}. \tag{9.4}$$

Step 3: Apply results for Poisson Accrual with minimum follow-up t = 0 to show that

$$\frac{\left(\frac{F_2}{dN_2} - Q\right)}{V_2} \xrightarrow{D} N(0, 1),$$

where

$$V_2^2 = \frac{Q^2}{As\ e^{-Qt}} \left[1 - \frac{1}{(dQs)}\left\{1 - e^{-dQs}\right\}\right]^{-1}$$

$$= \frac{Q}{dE(N_2)}. \tag{9.5}$$

This distribution holds independently of that of Step 2.

NOTE ON STEP 3: From the appendix on Poisson Processes, since patients must survive at least t to accrue time past t, arrivals past time t is a Poisson process with arrival rate

$$Ae^{-Qt} = A\ P[\text{Survival at least } t].$$

The "clock" for this process starts at calendar time t.

Step 4: Based on the already established results,

$$\frac{N_1}{E(N_1)} \xrightarrow{P} 1$$

and

$$\frac{N_2}{E(N_2)} \xrightarrow{P} 1.$$

Step 5: Show that

$$\frac{Q^* - Q}{V} \xrightarrow{D} N(0, 1)$$

where

$$Q^* = \frac{V_2^2}{V_1^2 + V_2^2}\left(\frac{F_1}{N_1}\right) + \frac{V_1^2}{\left(V_1^2 + V_2^2\right)}\left(\frac{F_2}{dN_2}\right)$$

and V^2, V_1^2, and V_2^2 are given in (9.2), (9.4), and (9.5) respectively.

Step 6: Apply Step 4 and Slutzky's Theorem to show

$$\frac{\hat{Q} - Q}{V} \xrightarrow{D} N(0, 1).$$

Footnote:

It is readily seen that

$$V^2 = \left(\frac{1}{V_1^2} + \frac{1}{V_2^2}\right)^{-1}$$

$$= \left(\frac{E(N_1)}{Q} + \frac{dE(N_2)}{Q}\right)^{-1} \qquad (9.6)$$

Now from (5.10),and Step 1 of Section 3.5

$$E(N_1) = \frac{E(F_1)}{Q}$$

and

$$E(N_2) = \frac{E(F_2)}{dQ}$$

Thus,

$$V^2 = \left(\frac{E(F_1) + E(F_2)}{Q^2}\right)^{-1} = \frac{Q^2}{\text{Expected Failures}}$$

for this reason, power is connected by many authors to the expected number of failures. If one has proportional hazards, and the expected number of failures per group is fixed, exponentiality is not a factor in the power of the logrank test.

Sample Size Equation for Poisson Accrual and Piecewise Exponential Survival:

Two sample trial with 50% allocation to each treatment. One-Sided Test Calculation (Replace α by $\alpha/2$ for Two-Sided Test.)

$$\frac{B^2 + C^2}{(.5As)} = \frac{(Q - T)^2}{(Z_\alpha + Z_\beta)^2} \qquad (9.7)$$

A = Total accrual rate. (.5A to each treatment).

s = Total calendar time of accrual

t = Time from end of accrual to analysis (minimum follow-up time).

d = Hazard rate after t: Hazard Rate Before t (ratio) (FACT in Sample Size Program)

Q = Daily failure rate on Treatment #1 (under H_A) to time t.

T = Daily failure rate on Treatment #2 (under H_A) to time t.

α = Probability of a Type I error (Reject H_0 when true).

Z_α = Upper 100α% point of the standard normal distribution.

β = 1 - Power = Probability of a Type II error (Reject H_A when true).

Z_β = Upper 100β% point of the standard normal

$$B^2 = \frac{Q^2}{As}\left[1 - \frac{e^{-Qt}}{(dQs)}\left\{1 - e^{-dQs}\right\}\right]^{-1}. \tag{9.8}$$

$$C^2 = \frac{T^2}{As}\left[1 - \frac{e^{-Tt}}{(dTs)}\left\{1 - e^{-dTs}\right\}\right]^{-1}. \tag{9.9}$$

See Section 3.10 regarding losses to follow-up.

Typical values for this Piecewise Exponential are

d = "FACT" = 0 (up front accrual) $\left(\lim_{d \to 0}\right)^*$

= .25 (75% hazard reduction)

= .50 (50% hazard reduction)

= .75 (25% hazard reduction)

= 1.00 exponential.

Increased hazard after t is not expected in any real clinical trial.

(* See (9.2) and (9.3))

3.10 Losses to Follow-Up and Sample Size Adjustment

The calculations of our sample size formulas assume no losses to follow-up (completing losses). (Patients quitting the study or failing due to non-study related cause are "lost to follow-up".)

The validity of a trial can be compromised by such losses, unless that are "uninformative." (Rubinstein et al. (1981) provide a formal method to adjust for such uninformative losses to follow-up.) We shall employ a less formal approach.

If a loss is uninformative, then the prognosis of the patient, given the treatment and time of removal from follow-up is presumed to be identical to patients, who stay on study and who are on that treatment, from the corresponding time onward.

EXAMPLE 10.1

A patient, who has completed therapy, moves with her parents to a region where follow-up cannot be maintained. This patient had been followed for 27 months, and was on Treatment #2. This seems to be an uninformative loss to follow-up. It seems reasonable to believe that the patient's prognosis has not been altered by the move.

EXAMPLE 10.2

In a study of coronary heart disease (CHD) a patient on Treatment #2 died at 25 months from a Non-CHD cause. If the major analysis is to be based on CHD events, then this patient is censored at 25 months. The patient would be counted in all days prior to death and would not be considered a CHD failure. We are forced to assume that the loss is uninformative, but this might not be a valid assumption. For example, if the patient died of renal failure, it might be indicative of poor vascular function. The CHD outlook of such a patient, assuming that the patient had survived the renal failure, might be much worse than other patients.

In clinical trials, site specific endpoints are especially prone to bias caused by competing losses. If one treatment has a greater tendency for such losses than the other, it might be difficult or impossible to interpret the results of the trial. Even in studying mortality, if one treatment is more toxic than the other, that treatment may lose more patients to follow-up than the other, compromising the trial.

Aggressive follow-up is a requirement of all clinical trials. External references can help keep track of participants. The National Death Index (National Center for Health Statistics) can help identify which losses have survived or died, provided that proper identifiers are collected.

For planning a study, although losses to follow-up are included in the analysis up to the time they leave the study, and therefore in theory reduce the variance of the statistics, it is recommended that the study be planned as if these patients contribute nothing. This is a bit conservative if losses are indeed uninformative.

Adjustment for Losses to Follow-Up

Let

N_u = Sample Size obtained from the Program (Unadjusted).

Based on the length of time needed to accrue N_u patients let

L = Fraction of patients expected to be lost to follow-up.

Then the adjusted sample size is

$$N_A = \frac{N_u}{1 - L}.$$

For example, if

$$N_u = 513$$

$$L = .1 \qquad \text{(10\% to be lost to follow-up)}$$

$$N_A = \frac{513}{1 - .1} = \frac{513}{.9} = 570$$

The recommended trial size is 570.

3.11 Interpretation of the Program

The sample sizes are obtained from (9.7) for Poisson Accrual, (7.1) for Up Front Accrual, and A133 for the Kaplan-Meier (Binomial). A computer routine readily solves (9.7) and (7.1) by bisection.

The parameters for the Program are identified with (9.7) and (7.1) as follows (the term minimum follow-up is t, the planned endpoint).

(a) Expected Accrual Through Minimum Follow-up = At

= (Accrual Rate)(Minimum Follow-up).

(b) PCONT $= e^{-tQ}$ (t = endpoint duration in days) (Q under H_A)

= Control Anticipated Survival Rate at time t, under H_A.

(c) DEL $= e^{-tT} - e^{-tQ}$ (T, Q under H_A)

= Difference between anticipated survival rates at time t

(d) ALPHA = α. (If two-sided, replace α by $\alpha/2$).

(e) POWER = 1 - β.

(f) FACT = d

= Hazard rate after t: Hazard rate before t.

3.12 Multi-Treatment Trials (3+ Treatments)

NOTE: This section reflects the majority position among statisticians, but is not universally accepted.

Generally, there are several types of multi-treatment trials, with different objectives. We shall discuss the four most common. It is rarely practical to use more than three or four treatments.

3.12.1 Type A

The treatments in this type of trial are generally as follows: (3 treatment case)

Control

Control + X

Control + Y

The experimental questions are:

(1) Is X efficacious?

(2) Is Y efficacious?

In this trial, assume that comparison of (Control + X) versus (Control + Y) is not a primary objective.

This type of trial would be conducted to learn what component of therapy may have efficacy. Hopefully, this experience will lead to a future trial, incorporating one or both of X and Y.

This type of trial should be designed exactly as a two treatment trial, except that the accrual per comparison is only two thirds that of a two treatment study.

$$\text{ACCRUAL THROUGH minimum follow-up} = \text{Atx} \tag{12.1}$$

A = Annual Accrual Rate.

t = Minimum Follow-up (Endpoint).

$$x = \frac{2}{\text{Number of Treatments}}. \qquad \text{(2/3 in our case)}$$

The analysis would compare Control versus Control + X by a one-sided logrank test and Control versus Control + Y by a one-sided logrank test.

<u>Controversy:</u> Some statisticians insist on controlling the overall error rate of the study, by adjusting

the P-Value through a formal "multiple comparison" procedure. We believe that such adjustment is not appropriate for the stated objectives of the trial, however.

- Had you done the two trials sequentially

Control	versus	Control + X	(Trial 1)
Control	versus	Control + Y	(Trial 2)

you would not have made such an adjustment.

- Why should data on the Control + Y group influence the efficacy comparison involving X?

3.12.2 Type B

The treatments for this type of trial are generally as follows: (3 treatment case).

Control

Control + X

Control + X + Y

The experimental questions are

(1) Is X efficacious?

(2) Is Y efficacious over and above X?

Here, the only adjustment centers around the accrual rate, which is handled as in Type A.

The following numerical example might be helpful.

Accrual Rate:	150 patients per year
Planning two year survival:	40% (Control)
	55% (Control + X)
	65% (Control + X + Y)

FACT = .50 (Post two year hazard = 50% of Pre two-year hazard)

ALPHA = .05 (one-sided)

POWER = .80

MINIMUM FOLLOW-UP = 2 years

Effective Accrual Rate = 100 per comparison per year (200 through minimum follow-up)

From the program, assuming negligible losses to follow-up we have:

Sample Size: 231 (Control versus Control + X)

437 (Control + X versus Control + X + Y)

In practice, we would run the trial as follows:

- Three-way randomization until 231 patients on Control or Control + X.
- Two-way randomization thereafter, with no controls. The first question will only utilize the 231 Control versus Control + X patients accrued in the three-way randomization.

In terms of total accrual time, at 150 patients per year, the three-way randomization would take about 2.3 years to accrue 346 patients (231 to question 1). It would take about 1.4 years to accrue the remaining 206 patients to answer the second question.

Technical Note: The accrual to the second experimental question was not Poisson, but skewed slightly toward later accrual. Thus it might be instructive to look at the second question assuming a two-way randomization throughout. (Accrual of 300 patients through the minimum follow-up.) This would require a sample of 467 (rather than 437). The actual trial has a greater expected follow-up than this hypothetical trial. Purists can either extend accrual by 30 in the two-way randomization, or extend follow-up about three additional months on the actual setup to achieve the power objective.

3.12.3 Type C: (All Two-Way Comparisons) The experimental questions here are

(1) Is there a difference between X and Y?

(2) Is there a difference between X and Z?

(3) Is there a difference between Y and Z?

If these are your questions and you are willing to treat these as three distinct trials, then the only adjustments that would be made would be

(a) Replace ALPHA by ALPHA/2. (two-sided tests)

(b) Effective accrual per comparison through minimum follow-up is two-thirds of the actual accrual through minimum follow-up.

However if you wish to find the best treatment, then multiple comparisons are needed. In fact, the concept of power changes. Our sample size program cannot be used to handle this situation, but can give conservative approximations.

The following example gives conservative sample sizes.

Annual Accrual: 225 per year (150 per comparison).

Minimum Follow-up: 2 years.

Two Year Survival: 50% versus 50% versus 70%.

FACT: 1.0 Exponential.

ALPHA: (.05)/3 = .0167 (two sided).

POWER: 90% (two specific comparisons with the best treatment).

You are going to infer that two treatments differ if the P-Value for comparing these treatments is less than .0167 (two-sided).

When there is in fact no difference between the treatments there is less than a 5% chance of falsely declaring a difference. (3 comparisons × .0167).

Your study will be successful if each comparison with the truly best treatment has a P-Value of below .0167 favoring the truly best treatment.

Since for each of the two comparisons with the truly best treatments there is a 10% chance of failing to declare superiority of the truly best treatment is at most a 20% chance of failing to declare the truly best treatment superior to one or both competitors. (At least 80% overall power to achieve your goal.)

Now the sample size is based on these parameters

$$Z_\alpha = 2.40 \qquad \text{(Figure 7)}$$

($Z_\alpha = 2.40$ corresponds to two-sided P-Value = .0167) and

$$Z_\beta = 1.28. \qquad \text{(Figure 6)}$$

Note that the sample size equation (9.7) depends on Z_α and Z_β only through their sum $Z_\alpha + Z_\beta$.

The following approximation greatly increases the use of the program:

Non-Utilized Z_α and Z_β

Actual $(Z_\alpha + Z_\beta) = U_A$

Utilized $(Z_\alpha + Z_\beta) = U_T$ (Fairly Close to U_A)

Sample Size from Program = N_T

Recommended Sample Size = N_A

$$N_A = N_T \frac{U_A^2}{U_T^2} \qquad (12.2)$$

This approximation is evident in (7.1) and (9.7).

For our program we have

ALPHA	POWER	BETA	$(Z_\alpha + Z_\beta) = U_T$
.005	.8	.20	3.42
.005	.9	.10	3.86
.01	.8	.20	3.17
.01	.9	.10	3.61
.025	.8	.20	2.80
.025	.9	.10	3.24
.05	.8	.20	2.48
.05	.9	.10	2.92

In the actual application,

$$U_A = 2.40 + 1.28 = 3.68.$$

This yields for ACCRUAL THROUGH MINIMUM FOLLOW-UP of 300, PCONT = .50, DEL = .20, FACT = 1.0, ALPHA = .01, and POWER = .9, a sample size of $N_T = 252$ per comparison (126 per treatment). From (12.2)

$$N_A = \frac{(3.68)^2\ 252}{(3.61)^2} = 262.$$

That is, 131 patients per treatment are required for a total of 393.

3.12.4 Type D: (2 × 2 Factorial Design) This is designed as follows:

Control

Control + X

Control + Y

Control + X + Y

The major therapeutic questions are usually

(1) Is X efficacious?

(2) Is Y efficacious?

Generally speaking, if one is willing to assume that no "qualitative interaction" between X and Y exists, then you can collapse this to two two-treatment questions. That is, if you believe that if X is efficacious, it will be efficacious whether or not Y is used, you may pool the groups without X and the groups with X for the comparison, (assuming that the randomization is about 25% to each treatment). Most statisticians would "stratify" the analysis as discussed in Section 3.13.

X Comparison: (Control) and (Control + Y) versus (Control + X) and (Control + X + Y)

Y Comparison: (Control) and (Control + X) versus (Control + Y) and (Control + X + Y)

In the absence of qualitative interaction, the Type D trial allows you to answer two questions for the price of one.

A test for Qualitative Interaction appears in Gail and Simon(1985).

3.13 Stratified Logrank Test

Often in clinical trials, investigators worry about imbalance in important prognostic groups. For example, it may be known that the extent of disease at baseline, as measured by lesion size, is highly predictive of outcome. Lesions below 5 cm in diameter have excellent prognosis, while lesions over 10 cm in diameter have a terrible prognosis.

The trial can be conducted in two ways: Prospective Stratification or Retrospective Stratification.

(A) Prospective Stratification

Conduct the study as if three trials were going on. Each trial will assign about equal numbers of patients to each treatment. Populations for Trials 1, 2, and 3 are respectively.

Stratum 1: Patients with lesions less than 5 cm in diameter.

Stratum 2: Patients with lesions 5 - 10 cm in diameter.

Stratum 3: Patients with lesions over 10 cm in diameter.

The analysis for comparing outcomes in a two treatment trial is as follows: (Illustration for three strata.)

Stratum	Observed Failures on Treatment #1	Expected Failures on Treatment #1	Variance
1	O_1	X_1	V_1
2	O_2	X_2	V_2
3	O_3	X_3	V_3
Total	O_T	X_T	V_T

$$Z = \frac{O_T - X_T}{\sqrt{V_T}} \tag{13.1}$$

The P-Value is obtained from the standard normal table (Figure 6 or Figure 7) depending upon whether the comparison is one-sided or two-sided.

> In summary, add the observed failures on Treatment #1 (O_T), the expected failures on Treatment #1 (X_T), and the variances (V_T). Compute Z as per (13.1) and determine the approximate P-Value from Figure 6 or Figure 7.

NOTE: As long as the number of strata is fairly small relative to the number of patients, prospective stratification has minimal impact on sample size requirements.

The sample sizes of this volume should be viewed as slightly conservative for use in prospectively stratified trials. That is, the sample size calculation slightly overestimates the true needs, since prospective stratification creates greater risk factor homogeneity between the groups than could be expected by chance. However, if the trial was conducted as a randomized study without using prospective stratification, the stratum specific percent of patients assigned to each treatment will still approach 50% as the sample size increases to infinity. In other words, for large trials with few strata, the benefit of stratification is more psychological than real.

(B) Retrospective Stratification

Patients would be randomized as if the trial was not stratified, but then the results would be analyzed as if the trial was stratified. This is a perfectly valid procedure. In practice, with a large sample size and few retrospective strata, the sample size requirements for the post stratified analysis are slightly less than those obtained in the program, and slightly more than the Prospectively Stratified Trial. The sample sizes are therefore conservative, but only slightly so.

Retrospective Stratification is very useful for exploratory analysis. For example, if you conduct a trial and discover that the two treatment groups have a serious imbalance in an important prognostic category, you may wish to rerun the analysis, adjusting for this imbalance via retrospective stratification. If this analysis qualitatively agrees with the planned analysis, then the final results are supported. However, in the rare case that they disagree, the analysis still provides important insight as to an explanation of the difference or lack of a difference between the treatments.

3.13.1 ADVICE ON STRATIFICATION

1. If used at all, limit the number of strata to a small number. When you stratify, the efficacy comparison only compares patients within the same strata.

The following is illustrative

Stratum 1:	10 patients assigned to Treatment #1
	10 patients assigned to Treatment #2
Stratum 2:	10 patients assigned to Treatment #1
	10 patients assigned to Treatment #2

In the stratified trial, the outcome of each Treatment #1 patient is compared to only 10 Treatment #2 patients, while the unstratified trial has 20 Treatment #2 patients to compare with each Treatment #1 patient. If you overstratify, the lack of ability to compare more than offsets the homogeneity created.

2. If you have stratum specific therapeutic questions, you must calculate sample size needs for each stratum separately. This could lead to a very much larger trial, than one where stratification is used only as a balancing tool.

3. If limited stratification is used to balance the randomization, the sample size requirements will be well approximated by the program, derived for non-stratified studies.

3.14 Intuitive Justification Why the Logrank Test and Kaplan-Meier Estimation for Actual Accrual Process Behave in the Limit in the Same Way as the Fixed Binomial Assumption

Consider the distribution on Day j given the history of the trial up to day j. In other words, if we had the trial results for all patients' day 1, day 2, ..., day j-1, we would know N_j and M_j the number of patients at risk at the start of day j. Given this information, F_j and G_j are binomial with respective sample sizes N_j and M_j and respective failure rates Q_j and T_j. This <u>conditional</u> distribution is identical to the unconditional distribution of the fixed binomial case.

$$E\left(\frac{F_j}{N_j} \mid \text{Past History of Trial}\right) = Q_j \qquad (N_j \neq 0)$$

$$\text{Var}\left(\frac{F_j}{N_j} \mid \text{Past History of Trial}\right) = \frac{Q_j P_j}{N_j} \qquad (N_j \neq 0)$$

As an estimate of Q_j, if we can ignore the possibility that $N_j = 0$, we can say, F_j/N_j is unbiased for Q_j and is uncorrelated with its past history.

Consider an alternate trial where we shall preselect N_j as

$$N_j^* = E(N_j) \qquad \text{(rounded to an integer)}$$

If $N_j \geq N_j^*$ we shall use the actual first N_j^* day j's of the trial.

If $N_j \leq N_j^*$ we shall add an additional $(N_j^* - N_j)$ day j's (independent trials with failure rate Q_j).

Although it is difficult to prove at the mathematical level of this text, it is intuitively clear that $N_j/N_j^* \xrightarrow{P} 1$ as $N_j^* \to \infty$ and hence the <u>fraction</u> of overlapping data coverages to 100% as the $N_j^* \to \infty$.

In other words, it can be shown that the large sample distributions under the actual process and artificial fixed binomial accrual are identical. The non-overlapping data is an insignificant percentage.

3.15 Alternate Standard Error for the Kaplan-Meier Estimator

(Peto et al (1977))

The following estimator for D_k in 10 of the Notation chart of Chapter 3 is often used to obtain the standard error of the Kaplan-Meier estimator, $\hat{S}_k$.

$$D_k^* = \hat{S}_k\left\{(1 - \hat{S}_k)/N_{k+1}\right\}^{\frac{1}{2}} \tag{15.1}$$

This is not completely rigorous but has a number of desirable properties. Some intuitive justification will be shown below.

Advantages over Greenwood Formula (Notation Chart item 11).

(a) Can be computed from the Kaplan-Meier estimate at time k and the number of patients at risk at time k+1. It does not require a summation.

(b) It agrees well with the Greenwood Formula except in the right hand portion of the curve where the fraction censored is high.

(c) The standard error increases in the plateau portion of a curve as patients are censored. The Greenwood Formula has a standard error that changes only at times where failures occur. This leads to unrealistically low estimates of standard error by Greenwood's Formula for situations where few patients are at risk.

Disadvantages over Greenwood's Formula

(d) $\dfrac{\hat{S}_k - S_k}{D_k^*}$ is not in theory asymptotically standard normal. It is close to standard normal where the sample size is large and the fraction censored before k is small. We shall see in Theorem 15.1 that the use of D_k^* is conservative $(\hat{D}_k \leq D_k^*)$.

(e) If one wishes to make statements such as "We are 95% confident that the three year survival is less than x", then the Greenwood standard error is superior, even in plateaus. This is because survival curves are monotonically decreasing functions. Hence, if you are 95% confident that the two year survival is below 83%, you are certainly 95% confident that the three year survival is below 83%, whether or not there is a large fraction of patients censored between two and three years. If the two to three year interval is a plateau, for example, the upper limit of the 95% confidence interval for the alternate standard error will be higher at three years than at two years, while that of Greenwood's formula will remain fixed.

Intuitive justification of the alternative standard error:

Theorem 15.1: $D_k^* \geq \hat{D}_k$

Proof: From item 9 of the Notation Chart at the beginning of Chapter 3,

$$1 - \hat{S}_k = 1 - \prod_{j=1}^{k} \hat{P}_j. \tag{15.2}$$

Now, by applying the lemma on converting a difference of products to a sum (Section 3.2) with

$$a_j = 1 \quad \text{and } b_j = \hat{P}_j,$$

we have

$$1 - \hat{S}_k = \hat{S}_k \sum \frac{(1-\hat{P}_j)}{\hat{S}_j}$$

$$= \hat{S}_k \sum \frac{\hat{Q}_j}{\hat{S}_{j-1}\hat{P}_j}. \tag{15.3}$$

Now,

$$\frac{\hat{S}_k}{\hat{S}_{j-1}} = \frac{\hat{P}_1 \cdots \hat{P}_k}{\hat{P}_1 \cdots \hat{P}_{j-1}} = \hat{P}_j \cdots \hat{P}_k. \tag{15.4}$$

Now from the <u>actual</u> accrual process,

$$N_{j+1} = N_j - F_j - W_j$$

where

N_j = Number of Patients at risk at start of day j,

F_j = Failures on Day j,

W_j = Competing "withdrawals" on Day j.

The W_j include patients who are alive with time of risk j, as well as those who quit alive on day j.

$$\hat{P}_j = \frac{N_j - F_j}{N_j} \geq \frac{N_j - F_j - W_j}{N_j} = \frac{N_{j+1}}{N_j}. \tag{15.5}$$

As long as the W_j are small percentages of N_j, approximate equality holds.

By substituting (15.5) into (15.4) we have

$$\frac{\hat{S}_k}{\hat{S}_{j-1}} \geq \prod_{i=j}^{k} \frac{N_{i+1}}{N_i} = \frac{N_{k+1}}{N_j}. \tag{15.6}$$

Substituting (15.6) in (15.3) yields

$$1 - \hat{S}_k \geq N_{k+1} \sum_j \frac{\hat{Q}_j}{N_j \hat{P}_j}. \tag{15.7}$$

Hence

$$\frac{(1 - \hat{S}_k)}{N_{k+1}} \geq \sum_j \frac{\hat{Q}_j}{N_j \hat{P}_j}. \tag{15.8}$$

That is,

$$D_k^* = \hat{S}_k\left\{\frac{(1 - \hat{S}_k)}{N_{k+1}}\right\}^{\frac{1}{2}}$$

$$\geq \hat{D}_k = \hat{S}_k\left\{\sum \frac{\hat{Q}_j}{N_j\hat{P}_j}\right\}^{\frac{1}{2}} \tag{15.9}$$

and approximate equality holds as long as the withdrawal rates are small fractions of the N_j.

Summary:

The use of D_k^* instead of $\hat{D}_k$ is conservative. The formula will underestimate the precision of the estimator $\hat{S}_k$, but only slightly if the fraction of competing withdrawals is small.

3.16 Connection Between Kaplan-Meier and Binomial

Note that if there are no censored patients to day k, under actual accrual, $N_{j+1} = N_j - F_j$ and

$$\hat{P}_j = \frac{N_{j+1}}{N_j}.$$

This yields from the Notation Chart:

$$\hat{S}_k = \prod_{j=1}^{k} \frac{N_{j+1}}{N_j}$$

$$= \frac{N_2}{N_1}\frac{N_3}{N_2}\cdots\frac{N_{k+1}}{N_k} = \frac{N_{k+1}}{N_1}. \tag{16.1}$$

To evaluate $\hat{D}_k^2$, note that

$$\hat{Q}_j = 1 - \hat{P}_j = \frac{N_j - N_{j+1}}{N_j}$$

and hence

$$\frac{\hat{Q}_j}{\hat{P}_j N_j} = \frac{N_j - N_{j+1}}{N_{j+1} N_j} = \frac{1}{N_{j+1}} - \frac{1}{N_j}$$

$$\sum_{j=1}^{k} \frac{\hat{Q}_j}{\hat{P}_j N_j} = \sum_{j=1}^{k} \left(\frac{1}{N_{j+1}} - \frac{1}{N_j} \right)$$

$$= \left(\frac{1}{N_2} - \frac{1}{N_1} \right) + \left(\frac{1}{N_3} - \frac{1}{N_2} \right) + \cdots + \left(\frac{1}{N_{k+1}} - \frac{1}{N_k} \right)$$

$$= \frac{1}{N_{k+1}} - \frac{1}{N_1} = \frac{N_1 - N_{k+1}}{N_1 N_{k+1}}$$

Hence

$$\hat{D}_k^2 = \hat{S}_k^2 \sum_{j=1}^{k} \frac{\hat{Q}_j}{\hat{P}_j N_j}$$

$$= \frac{N_{k+1}^2}{N_1^2} \frac{(N_1 - N_{k+1})}{N_1 N_{k+1}}$$

$$= \frac{N_{k+1}(N_1 - N_{k+1})}{N_1^3}$$

$$= \frac{\hat{S}_k(1 - \hat{S}_k)}{N_1} \qquad (16.2)$$

$\hat{D}_k^2$ is the binomial estimate of variance when there are no competing losses.

Studies based on the Kaplan-Meier are planned using the Binomial output (program). Adjustments can be made for anticipated losses to follow-up. (See **A133** for details).

REFERENCES

1. **Crowley, J.**, Asymptotic normality of a new nonparameteric statistic for use in organ transplant studies, *J. Am. Statist. Assoc.,* 69, 1006, 1974.
2. **Breslow, N.E.** and **Crowley, J.**, A large sample study of the life table and product limit estimates under random censorship, *Ann. Statist.* 2, 437, 1974.
3. **Gail, M.** and **Simon, R.**, Testing for qualitative interaction between treatment effects and patient subsets, *Biometrics,* 41, 362, 1985.

4. **Greenwood, M.,** *The Errors of Sampling of the Survivorship Tables, Reports on Public Health and Statistical Subjects,* Her Majesty's Stationery Office, London, 1926, 33.

5. **Kaplan, E. L. and Meier, P.,** Nonparametric estimation from incomplete observations, *J. Am. Statist. Assoc.*, 53, 447, 1958.

6. **Peto, R., Pike, M. C., Armitage, P., Breslow, N. E., Cox, D. R., Howard, S. V., Mantel, N., McPherson, K., Peto, J., and Smith, P. G.,** Design and analysis of randomized clinical trials requiring prolonged observation of each patient, II. Analysis and example, *Br. J. Canc.*, 35, 1, 1977.

7. **Rubinstein, L. V., Gail, M. H., and Santner, T. J.,** Planning the duration of a comparitive clinical trial with loss to follow-up and a period of continued observation, *J. Chron. Dis.*, 34, 469, 1981.

APPENDIX I

A REVIEW OF MATHEMATICAL STATISTICS

In order to follow the material in Chapter 3, it is assumed that the reader has a working knowledge of undergraduate mathematical statistics at a level of one of the following texts: Mendenhall, Scheaffer, and Wackerly (1986), Fraser (1976), Mood, Graybill, and Boes (1974), or Hogg and Craig (1978).

In order that this book be self contained, this appendix will list definitions and results. For convenient reference each is assigned a number.

A.1 Sample Space(s) (Definition): The set of all possible outcomes of an experiment (study or observation process). This is denoted by S.

A.2 Event (Definition): A subset of the Sample Space.

A.3 Union of Events: $E_1 \cup E_2$ (Definition) An event consisting of outcomes in one or both of E_1, E_2. (Unites the two events into a larger event).

This definition extends to multi-events $E_1 \cup E_2 \cup E_3$ etc.

A.4 Intersection of Events: E_1E_2 (Definition) An event consisting of outcomes common to E_1 and E_2. To qualify for membership in E_1E_2, the outcome must be in both event E_1 and event E_2.

This definition extends to multi-events $E_1E_2E_3$ etc.

A.5 Complement of Event: $(\bar{E})$ (Definition) The complement of the event E, denoted by $\bar{E}$, consists of all outcomes in the sample space that are not in the event E. (E and $\bar{E}$ have no outcomes in common, and together make up the sample space $E \cup \bar{E} = S$).

A.6 Null Event: $(\emptyset)$ (Definition) The Event which contains no outcomes in the sample space is called the null Event $(\emptyset = \bar{S})$.

A.7 Mutually Exclusive Events (Definition): The events E_1 and E_2 are mutually exclusive if they have no outcomes in common. $E_1E_2 = \emptyset$.

This definition extends to multi-events $E_1, E_2, \ldots, E_n$ as $E_iE_j = \emptyset$ for every i,j $1 \leq i < j \leq n$.

A.8 Probability (Definition) P is called a probability if

(a) P assigns a number P(E) to every event in S with $0 \leq P(E) \leq 1$.

(b) If $E_1, E_2, \ldots, E_n$ are mutually exclusive events $P(E_1 \cup E_2 \cup \cdots \cup E_n) =$

$P(E_1)+P(E_2)+\cdots+P(E_n)$

(c) P(S) = 1 where S = Sample Space

Probability Results (Consequences)

A.9 (a) $P(\emptyset) = 0$

A.10 (b) $P(\bar{E}) = 1 - P(E)$

A.11 (c) $P(E_1 \cup E_2) = P(E_1) + P(E_2) - P(E_1 E_2)$

A.12 Conditional Probability $\left(P(E_1|E_2)\right)$ (Definition)

The probability that E_1 occurs given that E_2 has occurred is denoted by

$$P(E_1|E_2) = \frac{P(E_1 E_2)}{P(E_2)} \qquad \left(P(E_2) > 0\right)$$

A.13 Independence of two Events (Definition)

Events E_1 and E_2 are independent if $P(E_1 E_2) = P(E_1)P(E_2)$.

A.14 Independence of two events (Consequence)

Provided that $P(E_2)>0$, then events E_1 and E_2 are independent if and only if

$$P(E_1|E_2) = P(E_1)$$

i.e. conditional and unconditional probability agree.

The proof is straight forward and is therefore omitted.

A.15 Mutual Independence of Several Events (Definition)

Events $E_1, E_2, \ldots, E_n$ are mutually independent if for every subset $\left\{j_1, j_2, \ldots, j_k\right\}$ of the integers $\{1,2,\ldots,n\}$

$$P(E_{j_1} E_{j_2} \ldots E_{j_k}) = P(E_{j_1})P(E_{j_2}) \cdots P(E_{j_k})$$

A.16 Random Variable (Definition)

A random variable assigns a number to each outcome in the sample space S. That is, if X is a random variable, then for each sample point s in S, X assigns a number X(s).

A.17 Random Vector (Vector of Random Variables) (Definition)

A random vector, Y, of dimension k is a k-dimensional vector of random variables $(X_1,X_2,\ldots,X_k) = Y$

A.18 Cumulative Distribution Function of a Random Variable (cdf) (Definition)

The cumulative distribution function of the random variable X, denoted by $F_X(x)$, is

$$F_X(x) = P[X \leq x] \qquad -\infty < x < \infty$$

The cumulative distribution function is a plot of the probability that the random variable X takes on numerical value less than or equal to the number x. This is plotted over all real numbers, x.

A.19 Discrete Random Variables and Probability Mass Function (Definition)

A random variable X is "discrete" if the cumulative distribution is of the form

$$F_X(x) = \sum_{y:\, y \leq x} f_X(y)$$

y: $y \leq x$ refers to a finite set of possible values of the random variable X that assign values x or less and $F_X(x) \rightarrow 1$ as $x \rightarrow \infty$.

The function $f_X(y) = P[X=y]$ is called the probability mass function. This mass function will be zero except at a discrete set of values. (*This is not the most general definition, but it will meet our needs.*)

A.20 Continuous Random Variables and Probability Density Function (Definition)

A random variable X is "continuous" if the cumulative distribution is of the form

$$F_X(x) = \int_{-\infty}^{x} f_X(y)dy$$

with $F_X(x) \rightarrow 1$ as $x \rightarrow \infty$.

For the purpose of this volume, we shall assume that $f_X(y)$ has at most a finite number of discontinuities.

$f_X(y)$ is called the probability density function.

A.21 Relation between Cumulative Distribution and Probability Density Function (Consequence)

At each continuity point of $F_X(x)$,

$$f_X(x) = F'_X(x)$$

That is, the probability density is the derivative of the cumulative distribution function.

Proof: $$F_X(x+h) - F_X(x) = \int_x^{x+h} f_X(y)dy$$
$$= hf_X(\xi) \quad \text{for some } \xi\text{: } x \leq \xi \leq x+h$$

The above follows from the Mean Value Theorem of Calculus.

If we divide both sides by h and let $h \to 0$, the result follows.

A.22 Cumulative Distribution Function for Random Vectors (Definition)

We shall write this in terms of two random vectors, but the extension to several dimensions is clear.

A random vector $X = (X_1, X_2)$ has cumulative distribution denoted by F_X:

$$F_X(x_1,x_2) = P(X_1 \leq x_1, X_2 \leq x_2)$$

A.23 Multivariate Analogues of Mass Function and Density (Definition)

(a) X_1, X_2 discrete

$$f_X(x_1,x_2) = P[X_1 = x_1, X_2 = x_2]$$

$$F_X(x_1,x_2) = \sum_{\substack{y_1 \leq x_1 \\ y_2 \leq x_2}} f_X(y_1,y_2)$$

$f_X(x_1,x_2)$ is the joint probability mass function of X_1, X_2

(b) X_1, X_2 continuous

$$F_X(x_1,x_2) = \int_{-\infty}^{x_1}\int_{-\infty}^{x_2} f_X(y_1,y_2)dy_2dy_1$$

$f_X(x_1, x_2)$ is the joint probability density of X_1, X_2

Note: at continuity points of (x_1,x_2),

$$f_X(x_1,x_2) = \frac{\partial^2 F_X(x_1,x_2)}{\partial x_1 \partial x_2}$$

(c) X_1 discrete, X_2 continuous

$$F_X(x_1,x_2) = \sum_{y_1 \le x_1} \int_{-\infty}^{x_2} f_X(y_1,y_2)dy_2$$

$f_X(x_1,x_2)$ is the <u>joint probability mass-density</u> of X_1, X_2

A.24 <u>Marginal Distributions</u> (Definition and Consequences)

Here, we also study two variables X_1, X_2 but the extension to several variables is clear.

$$P[X_1 \le x_1] = \lim_{x_2 \to \infty} P[X_1 \le x_1, X_2 \le x_2]$$

$$= \lim_{x_2 \to \infty} F_X(x_1,x_2)$$

We denote this by the Marginal Cumulative Distribution of X_1:

$$F_{X_1}(x_1) = \lim_{x_2 \to \infty} F_X(x_1,x_2)$$

$$= \int_{-\infty}^{x_1} \left\{ \int_{-\infty}^{\infty} f_X(y_1,y_2)dy_2 \right\} dy_1 \qquad X_1,X_2 \text{ continuous}$$

$$= \sum_{y_1 \le x_1} \left\{ \sum_{\text{all } y_2} f_X(y_1,y_2) \right\} \qquad X_1,X_2 \text{ discrete}$$

$$= \sum_{y_1 \le x_1} \left\{ \int_{-\infty}^{\infty} f_X(y_1, y_2)dy_2 \right\} \qquad X_1 \text{ discrete, } X_2 \text{ continuous}$$

$$= \int_{-\infty}^{x_1} \left\{ \sum_{\text{all } y_2} f_X(y_1, y_2) \right\} dy_1 \qquad X_1 \text{ continuous, } X_2 \text{ discrete}$$

A25. If X_2 is <u>discrete</u>,

$$f_{X_1}(x_1) = \sum_{\text{all } y_2} f_X(x_1, y_2) \qquad \text{is}$$

called the <u>Marginal density of X_1</u> if X_1 is <u>continuous</u>, or <u>Marginal Mass function of X_1</u> if X_1 is <u>discrete</u>.

A26. If X_2 is continuous

$$f_{X_1}(x_1) = \int_{-\infty}^{\infty} f_X(x_1,y_2)dy_2 \quad \text{is}$$

called the Marginal density of X_1 if X_1 is continuous, or Marginal Mass function of X_1 if X_1 is discrete.

A27. Conditional Distributions (Definition and Consequences).

The Conditional Mass function (X_2 discrete) or conditional density (X_2 continuous) of X_2 given $X_1 = x_1$ is defined by

$$f_{X_2|X_1}(x_2|x_1) = \frac{f_X(x_1, x_2)}{f_{X_1}(x_1)}$$

If X_1 is continuous, the above definition only applies to continuity points of $f_{X_1}(x_1)$ and $f_X(x_1, x_2)$.

Notes: (a) If X_1 and X_2 are discrete, then by the definitions of conditional probability and marginal probability mass function (See A12 and A25)

$$f_{X_2|X_1}(x_2|x_1) = P[X_2 = x_2|X_1 = x_1]$$

(b) If X_1 and X_2 are continuous, (x_1, x_2) is a continuity point of f_X, and Δ_1 and Δ_2 are small:

$$P[x_1 < X_1 < x_1 + \Delta_1, x_2 < X_2 < x_2 + \Delta_2] \simeq \Delta_1\Delta_2 f_X(x_1, x_2)$$

$$P[x_1 < X_1 < x_1 + \Delta_1] \simeq \Delta_1 f_{X_1}(x_1)$$

$$P[x_2 < X_2 < x_2 + \Delta_2|x_1 < X_1 < x_1 + \Delta_1] \simeq \frac{\Delta_2 f_X(x_1, x_2)}{f_{X_1}(x_1)}$$

That is, in the limit, as $\Delta_1 \to 0$ and $\Delta_2 \to 0$,

$$f_{X_1|X_2}(x_2|x_1) = \frac{f_X(x_1, x_2)}{f_{X_1}(x_1)}$$

behaves as a density, reflecting the appropriate conditional probability.

(c) Similar analogues can be developed for mixed continuous-discrete random variables.

A28. Conditioning on an Event (consequence)

In the case of a continuous $X = (X_1, X_2)$ one may wish to find the conditional distribution of

X_2 given $X_1 < x_1$ rather than specifying an exact value of x_1.

$$P\left(X_2 < x_2|X_1 < x_1\right) = \frac{P\left[X_1 < x_1, X_2 < x_2\right]}{P\left[X_1 < x_1\right]}$$

$$= \frac{F_{X_1,X_2}(x_1, x_2)}{F_{X_1}(x_1)}$$

$$P\left[X_2 < x_2|X_1 < x_1\right] = \frac{\int_{-\infty}^{x_2}\left\{\int_{-\infty}^{x_1} f_X(y_1, y_2)dy_1\right\}dy_2}{F_{X_1}(x_1)}$$

This is the conditional cumulative distribution of X_2 given that $X_1 < x_1$.

Differentiating both sides with respect to x_2 yields the conditional density at continuity points:

$$f_{X_2|X_1}\left(x_2|X_1<x_1\right) = \frac{\int_{-\infty}^{x_1} f_X(y_1, x_2)dy_1}{F_{X_1}(x_1)}$$

A29. Independence of Random Variables (Definition)

Random variables X_1 and X_2 are independent if for every x_1, x_2

$$F_X(x_1, x_2) = F_{X_1}(x_1)F_{X_2}(x_2)$$

That is, for every x_1, x_2 the events

E_1 that	$X_1 \leq x_1$ and
E_2 that	$X_2 \leq x_2$ are independent.

A30. Independence of Random Variables (Consequence)

Independence is equivalent to

$$f_X(x_1, x_2) = f_{X_1}(x_1)f_{X_2}(x_2)$$

with f the mass or density function depending on whether the random variable is discrete or continuous.

The proofs are straight forward.

A31. Independence of Several Random Variables (Definition and Consequence)

Either of these definitions imply independence

$$\begin{aligned} F_X(x_1, x_2, \ldots, x_k) &= P[X_1 \leq x_1, X_2 \leq x_2, \ldots, X_k \leq x_k] \\ &= F_{X_1}(x_1)\, F_{X_2}(x_2) \ldots F_{X_k}(x_k) \quad \text{for all } (x_1, \ldots, x_k) \end{aligned}$$

or

$$f_X(x_1, \ldots, x_k) = f_{X_1}(x_1)\, f_{X_2}(x_2) \ldots f_{X_k}(x_k) \quad \text{for all } (x_1, \ldots, x_k)$$

A32. Random Samples (Independently Identically Distributed Random Variables) (IID random variables) (Definition)

Random variables $X_1, X_2, \ldots, X_k$ are independent identically distributed if they are independent and each X_j has the same cumulative distribution:

$$F_{X_j}(x) = F(x) \qquad \text{Same for all j.}$$

$$F_X(x_1, \ldots, x_k) = F(x_1)\, F(x_2) \ldots F(x_k)$$

or sufficiently

$$f_X(x_1, \ldots, x_k) = f(x_1)\, f(x_2) \ldots f(x_k).$$

EXPECTED VALUE OF A FUNCTION OF A RANDOM VECTOR (Definition)

A33. (a) Univariate

Let g(X) be a function of the random variable X. g(X) has expectation denoted by $E\big(g(X)\big)$

$$E\big(g(X)\big) = \int_{-\infty}^{\infty} g(x) f_X(x)dx \qquad \text{(Continuous Case)}$$

$$= \sum_{\text{all } x} g(x) f_X(x) \qquad \text{(Discrete case)}$$

f_X is the probability density for continuous X or the probability mass function for discrete X.

A34. (b) Multivariate

Let g(X) be a function of the random vector $X = (X_1, X_2)$. g(X) has expectation

$$E\big(g(X)\big) = \int_{-\infty}^{\infty}\int_{-\infty}^{\infty} g(x_1, x_2) f_X(x_1, x_2) dx_2 dx_1 \qquad \text{(Continuous case)}$$

with $f_X(x_1, x_2)$ the joint density of X_1. X_2.

Discrete components will involve sum instead of integral.

SPECIAL UNIVARIATE FUNCTIONS (Definitions)

We shall only write these for the continuous case, but they apply in similar fashion to the discrete case too.

A35. (a) $g(X) = X$ (The <u>population mean</u> of X)

We generally denote the mean by μ

$$\mu = E(X) = \int_{-\infty}^{\infty} x f_X(x) dx$$

A36. (b) $g(X) = (X-\mu)^2$ (The <u>population variance</u> of X)

We generally denote the population variance, the average squared deviation about the mean as σ^2

$$\begin{aligned} \text{Var}(X) &= E\left[(X-\mu)^2\right] \\ &= \int_{-\infty}^{\infty} (x-\mu)^2 f_X(x) dx \\ \text{where} \quad \mu &= E(X) \end{aligned}$$

A37. (c) $g(X) = e^{tX}$ (The <u>moment generating function</u> of X)

We generally denote this by $M_X(t)$

$$M_X(t) = \int_{-\infty}^{\infty} e^{tx} f_X(x)dx$$

A38. SPECIAL MULTIVARIATE FUNCTION

$$g(X) = (X_1 - \mu_1)(X_2 - \mu_2) \qquad \text{(Population Covariance)}$$

where $\mu_1 = E(X_1) \quad \mu_2 = E(X_2)$

$$\text{Cov}(X_1, X_2) = \int_{-\infty}^{\infty}\int_{-\infty}^{\infty} (x_1 - \mu_1)(x_2 - \mu_2) f_X(x_1, x_2) dx_2\, dx_1$$

RESULTS ON EXPECTATIONS (Consequences)

A39. (a) Expectation of a constant is a constant.

If $g(X) = C$ for all X,

$E\big(g(X)\big) = C$

A40. (b) If C is a constant,

$E\big(Cg(X)\big) = CE\big(g(X)\big)$

A41. (c) Additivity of Expectation

$E\{g_1(X) + g_2(X)\} = E\{g_1(X)\} + E\{g_2(X)\}$

A42. (d) $E\{\sum_{j=1}^{k} a_j g_j(X)\} = \Sigma a_j E\{g_j(X)\}$

A43. (e) Shortcut formula for Variance

$\sigma^2 = E\big((X-\mu)^2\big) = E(X^2) - \mu^2$

where $\mu = E(X)$

A44. (f) Shortcut formula for covariance

$$\mathrm{Cov}(X_1, X_2) = E\left\{(X_1-\mu_1)(X_2-\mu_2)\right\} \quad \text{(Definition)}$$

$$= E\left(X_1X_2\right)-\mu_1\mu_2 \quad \text{(Consequence)}$$

Proof (f)

$$(X_1 - \mu_1)(X_2-\mu_2) = X_1X_2-\mu_1X_2-\mu_2X_1 + \mu_1\mu_2$$

Take expectation on both sides and apply (d) and (a) above.

A45. (g) Linear Combinations (Consequence)

Let $Y = \sum_{j=1}^{k} a_jX_j$

Then $E(Y) = \sum_{j=1}^{k} a_j\mu_j$ where $\mu_j = E(X_j)$

and $\mathrm{Var}(Y) = \sum_{j=1}^{k} a_j^2\mathrm{Var}(X_j) + 2\sum_{j=2}^{k}\sum_{i=1}^{j-1} a_ia_j\mathrm{Cov}(X_i, X_j)$

Proof (g): The expectation of Y is obtained from (d) above.

$$\mathrm{Var}(Y) = E\left\{Y-E(Y)\right\}^2 = E\left(\left\{\sum_{j=1}^{k} a_j(X_j-\mu_j)\right\}^2\right)$$

= Desired Result by (d) above.

A46. (h) If X_1, X_2 are independent, then

$$\mathrm{Cov}\ (X_1, X_2) = 0$$

Proof (h):

$$E\left(X_1X_2\right) = \int_{-\infty}^{\infty}\int_{-\infty}^{\infty} x_1x_2f_X(x_1x_2)dx_2dx_1$$

$$= \int_{-\infty}^{\infty}\int_{-\infty}^{\infty} x_1x_2f_{X_1}(x_1)f_{X_2}(x_2)dx_2dx_1 \quad \text{(independence)}$$

$$= \int_{-\infty}^{\infty} x_1f_{X_1}(x_1)dx_1 \int_{-\infty}^{\infty} x_2f_{X_2}(x_2)dx_2$$

$$= \mu_1\mu_2$$

From (f) above, $\text{Cov}(X_1, X_2) = 0$

(i) Expectation and Variance for classical statistics for independent identically distributed random variables.

Let $X_1, X_2, \ldots, X_n$ be independent identically distributed random variables with

$$E(X_j) = \mu \quad \text{and} \quad \text{Var}(X_j) = \sigma^2$$

Let $\bar{X} = \dfrac{\sum_{j=1}^{n} X_j}{n}$ (Sample Mean)

$$S^2 = \frac{\sum_{j=1}^{n} (X_j - \bar{X})^2}{(n-1)} \qquad \text{(Sample Variance)}$$

A47. Then $E(\bar{X}) = \mu$

A48. $\text{Var}(\bar{X}) = \frac{\sigma^2}{n}$

A49. $E(S^2) = \sigma^2$

Proof (i): To prove the results for $\bar{X}$, we apply (g) above with $a_j = (\frac{1}{n})$. By independence $\text{Cov}(X_i, X_j) = 0$. This yields $E(\bar{X}) = \mu$ and $\text{Var}(\bar{X}) = \frac{\sigma^2}{n}$

$$S^2 = \frac{\left\{\Sigma X_j^2 - n\bar{X}^2\right\}}{(n-1)} \qquad (*)$$

From the shortcut formula

$\sigma^2 = E(X_j^2) - \mu^2$ implies $E(X_j^2) = \sigma^2 + \mu^2$

and $\text{Var}(\bar{X}) = E(\bar{X})^2 - \left\{E(\bar{X})\right\}^2$

i.e. $\frac{\sigma^2}{n} = E(\bar{X})^2 - \mu^2$.

Hence $E(\bar{X})^2 = \mu^2 + \frac{\sigma^2}{n}$.

Taking expectation in (*) yields:

$$E(S^2) = \frac{\{n\sigma^2 + n\mu^2 - n\mu^2 - \sigma^2\}}{(n-1)} = \sigma^2.$$

A50. (j) $|\mathrm{Cov}(X_1, X_2)| \leq \{\mathrm{Var}(X_1)\,\mathrm{Var}(X_2)\}^{\frac{1}{2}}.$

Proof (j): $\mathrm{Var}(X_1 + tX_2) = \mathrm{Var}(X_1) + 2t\,\mathrm{Cov}(X_1, X_2) + t^2\mathrm{Var}(X_2).$

Since Var ( ) ≥ 0, we obtain the result by successively letting $t = \pm\sqrt{\frac{\mathrm{Var}(X_1)}{\mathrm{Var}(X_2)}}.$

Note that this implies

$$-1 \leq \rho = \frac{\mathrm{Cov}(X_1, X_2)}{\{\mathrm{Var}(X_1)\,\mathrm{Var}(X_2)\}^{\frac{1}{2}}} \leq 1.$$

A51. (k) Chebyshev Theorem (Consequence)

Let X be a random variable with mean μ and variance σ^2. Then for any $\epsilon > 0$

$$P[|X-\mu| \geq \epsilon] \leq \frac{\sigma^2}{\epsilon^2}.$$

Proof: We shall prove the result in the continuous case

$$\begin{aligned}
\sigma^2 &= \int_{-\infty}^{\infty} (x-\mu)^2 f_X(x)dx \\
&\geq \int_{|x-\mu|\geq\epsilon} (x-\mu)^2 f_X(x)dx \\
&\geq \int_{|x-\mu|\geq\epsilon} \epsilon^2 f_X(x)dx \\
&\geq \epsilon^2 P[|X-\mu|\geq\epsilon].
\end{aligned}$$

Divide both sides by ϵ^2 to obtain the result.

A52. (l) "Consistency of $\bar{X}$" (Consequence)

If X_1, X_2, ... are independent, identically distributed random variables with mean μ and variance σ^2, then for any $\epsilon > 0$

$$P\left[|\bar{X}_n - \mu| > \epsilon\right] \to 0 \quad \text{as } n \to \infty$$

where $\bar{X}_n = \frac{\left(X_1 + \cdots + X_n\right)}{n}$.

In lay terms, this is the "Law of Averages".

Proof: From A47 and A48 above,

$$E(\bar{X}) = \mu \quad \text{and} \quad \text{Var}(\bar{X}) = \frac{\sigma^2}{n}.$$

By Chebyshev's Theorem (k)

$$P\left[|\bar{X} - \mu| > \epsilon\right] \leq \frac{\text{Var}(\bar{X})}{\epsilon^2} = \frac{\sigma^2}{n\epsilon^2} \to 0 \quad \text{as } n \to \infty.$$

MOMENT GENERATING FUNCTIONS (Consequences)

$$M_X(t) = E\left(e^{tX}\right)$$

A53. (a) If two cumulative distributions differ, then they have different moment generating functions. (The moment generating function uniquely identifies the distribution. In fact, we only need to identify the moment generating function in an open interval about t=0.)

See Fraser (1976, pages 544-546).

A54. (b) Provided the moment generating function is defined in a neighborhood of t = 0, then

$$E(X^n) = \lim_{t \to 0} M_X^{(n)}(t)$$

(The nth derivative of $M_X(t)$ with respect to t is taken, and then $t \to 0$.)

See Fraser (1976, page 233).

A55. (c) $M_X(t) = 1 + \sum_{j=1}^{\infty} \frac{E(X^j)t^j}{j!}$

See Fraser (1976, page 233).

A56. (d) If $X_1, X_2, \ldots, X_n$ are independent random variables with respective moment generating functions

$$M_{X_j}(t) \qquad j = 1, \ldots, n$$

and

$$Y = \sum_{j=1}^{n} a_j X_j$$

with a_j's constant. Then Y has moment generating function

$$M_Y(t) = \prod_{j=1}^{n} M_{X_j}(a_j t)$$

Proof (d):

$$e^{tY} = e^{t\Sigma a_j X_j} = \prod_{j=1}^{n} e^{t a_j X_j}$$

$$E(e^{tY}) = \prod_{j=1}^{n} E\left(e^{t a_j X_j}\right) \qquad \text{by independence}$$

$$= \prod_{j=1}^{n} M_{X_j}(a_j t) \qquad \text{by definition.}$$

SPECIAL DISTRIBUTIONS

BINOMIAL DISTRIBUTION (Discrete)

A57. (a) Probability Mass Function of the binomial distribution

$$f(x) = \binom{n}{x} p^x (1-p)^{n-x} \qquad x = 0, 1, \ldots, n \qquad 0<p<1$$

where
$$\binom{n}{x} = \frac{n!}{x!(n-x)!}$$

$$a! = a(a-1)\ldots 1$$

$$0! = 1$$

A58. (b) Mean and Variance

$\mu = np$

$\sigma^2 = np(1-p)$

A59. (c) Moment Generating Function

$$M_X(t) = \left\{pe^t + (1-p)\right\}^n$$

A60. (d) How it arises in the real world.

If X is the number of observed failures, in a sample of n independent trials, each with probability of failure, p, then X has the Binomial Probability Mass Function above.

POISSON DISTRIBUTION (Discrete)

A61. (a) Probability Mass Function **of the Poisson distribution.**

$$f(x) = \frac{\lambda^x e^{-\lambda}}{x!} \qquad x = 0,1,2,\ldots \qquad \lambda>0$$

A62. (b) Mean and Variance

$\mu = \lambda$

$\sigma^2 = \lambda$

A63. (c) Moment Generating Function

$$M_X(t) = \exp\left\{\lambda(e^t - 1)\right\}$$

A64. (d) How it arises in the real world.

Approximation to Binomial

If in the binomial, n is large and p is small with $np = \lambda$, then the Poisson distribution will provide an excellent approximation to the binomial distribution.

More formally, if $n \to \infty$ and $p \to 0$ with $np \to \lambda > 0$

$$\binom{n}{x} p^x (1-p)^{n-x} \to \frac{\lambda^x e^{-\lambda}}{x!} \qquad x = 0,1,2,\ldots$$

UNIFORM DISTRIBUTION (Continuous)

A65. (a) Probability Density Function of the uniform distribution.

$$f(x) = \frac{1}{B-A} \qquad A<x<B$$

A66. (b) Mean and Variance

$$\mu = (A+B)/2$$

$$\sigma^2 = (B-A)^2/12$$

A67. (c) Moment Generating Function

$$M_X(t) = \frac{1}{\{(B-A)t\}}\left\{e^{Bt} - e^{At}\right\}$$

A68. (d) How it arises in the real world

Roundoff error

A69. (e) Cumulative Distribution

$$F(x) = \frac{x-A}{B-A} \qquad A<x<B$$

EXPONENTIAL DISTRIBUTION (Continuous)

A70. (a) Probability Density Function of the exponential distribution

$$f(x) = \lambda e^{-\lambda x} \qquad x>0$$

A71. (b) Mean and Variance

$$\mu = (1/\lambda)$$

$$\sigma^2 = (1/\lambda)^2$$

A72. (c) Moment Generating Function

$$M_X(t) = \frac{\lambda}{\lambda-t} \qquad t<\lambda$$

A73. (d) How it arises in the real world

- As survival time data - see (f) below

A74. (e) Cumulative Distribution

$F(x) = 1 - e^{-\lambda x} \quad x>0$

A75. (f) Memoriless Property (Constant Hazard)

Let $s>0$ and $t>0$ and let X have the exponential distribution.

$P[X>t] = 1-F(t) = e^{-\lambda t}$

$$P[X>t+s|X>s] = \frac{P[X>t+s, X>s]}{P[X>s]}$$

$$= \frac{P[X>t+s]}{P[X>s]} = \frac{e^{-\lambda(t+s)}}{e^{-\lambda s}}$$

$$= e^{-\lambda t}$$

The exponential distribution would imply that an s-year old individual has the same outlook as a newborn, in terms of future life.

The "Hazard Rate" defined as

$$H(x) = \frac{f(x)}{1-F(x)} \quad x>0$$

$$= \frac{\lambda e^{-\lambda x}}{e^{-\lambda x}} = \lambda$$

$H(x)dx$ is the instantaneous probability of failure between x and x+dx, given survival of at least x.

A76. Constant Hazard implies exponentiality, since if

$$\frac{f(x)}{1-F(x)} = \lambda \qquad x>0$$

$$\int_0^t \frac{f(x)dx}{1-F(x)} = \lambda t$$

$$\log\left\{1-F(0)\right\} - \log\left\{1-F(t)\right\} = \lambda t$$

Now $F(0) = 0$ for a survival distribution, and hence

$$1-F(t) = e^{-\lambda t}$$

GAMMA DISTRIBUTION (Continuous)

A77. (a) Probability Density of gamma distribution.

$$f(x) = \frac{\lambda^{\alpha} x^{\alpha-1} e^{-\lambda x}}{\Gamma(\alpha)} \qquad x>0,\ \alpha>0,\ \lambda>0$$

$$\Gamma(\alpha) = \int_0^{\infty} x^{\alpha-1} e^{-x} dx$$

Note: if α is an integer, n

$$\Gamma(n) = (n-1)!$$

A78. (b) Mean and Variance

$$\mu = (\alpha/\lambda)$$

$$\sigma^2 = (\alpha/\lambda^2)$$

A79. (c) Moment Generating Function

$$M_X(t) = \left\{\lambda/(\lambda-t)\right\}^{\alpha} \qquad t<\lambda$$

A80. (d) How it arises in the real world

- If α=1, note that we obtain the exponential distribution

- Let $X_1, X_2, \ldots, X_n$ be independent, identically distributed exponential random variables with parameter λ.

Let $S = X_1 + X_2 + \cdots + X_n$

Then S has the Gamma Distribution with parameters α=n and λ.

Proof From A72 and A56, S has moment generating function

$$M_S(t) = M_{X_1}(t)\, M_{X_2}(t) \dots M_{X_n}(t)$$

$$= \left\{\frac{\lambda}{(\lambda - t)}\right\}^n.$$

From the uniqueness property of Moment Generating Functions A53, and by A79, the result holds.

A81. The "chi-square" Distributions are special Gamma Distributions with

$\alpha = \text{(Degrees of Freedom)}/2$

$\lambda = \frac{1}{2}$

A82. (e) Cumulative Distribution (Integer α only)

Let $\alpha = n$ (an integer)

$$F(x) = 1 - \sum_{j=0}^{n-1} \frac{(\lambda x)^j e^{-\lambda x}}{j!}$$

Proof Differentiation of both sides yields result. (See A21.).

Note: Clear cut connection between Poisson Distribution and Gamma Distribution.

NORMAL DISTRIBUTION (Continuous)

A83. (a) Probability Density of normal distribution

$$f(x) = \frac{1}{\sigma\sqrt{2\pi}} \exp\left\{-(x-\mu)^2/2\sigma^2\right\} \qquad -\infty < x < \infty$$

A84. (b) Mean and Variance

We have so denoted the two parameters μ and σ^2 ($\pi = 3.1416$).

A85. (c) Moment Generating Function

$$M_X(t) = \exp\left(\mu t + \tfrac{1}{2}\sigma^2 t^2\right)$$

A86. (d) Cumulative Distribution

No closed form, but the usual notation is

$F(x) = \Phi\left(\frac{x-\mu}{\sigma}\right)$ with

$\Phi(t) = \int_{-\infty}^{t} \frac{1}{\sqrt{2\pi}} \exp(-t^2/2)dt$

Φ is called the "Standard Normal" cumulative distribution, often denoted by N(0,1).

A87. (e) Difference of independent normal random variables is normal.

Let X_1, X_2, be independent normally disributed random variables with respective means μ_1 and μ_2 and respective variances σ_1^2 and σ_2^2. Then $(X_1 - X_2)$ is normal with mean μ_1-μ_2 and variance $\sigma_1^2+\sigma_2^2$.

Proof:

$$E\left(e^{t(X_1-X_2)}\right) = E(e^{tX_1})E(e^{-tX_2}) \qquad \text{Independence}$$

$$= \exp\left(\mu_1 t + \tfrac{1}{2}\sigma_1^2 t^2\right) \exp\left(-\mu_2 t + \tfrac{1}{2}\sigma_2^2 t^2\right) \qquad \text{by (c)}$$

$$= \exp\left\{(\mu_1-\mu_2)t + \tfrac{1}{2}(\sigma_1^2+\sigma_2^2)t^2\right\}$$

X_1-X_2 has the moment generating function of a normal random variable with mean $(\mu_1$-$\mu_2)$ and variance $\sigma_1^2 + \sigma_1^2$. The result follows from A53.

A88 (f) How it arises in the real world.

-The Central Limit Theorem

Let $X_1, X_2, \ldots, X_n$, be a sequence of independent, identically distributed random variables with mean μ and variance σ^2. Let $\bar{X}_n = (X_1 + \cdots + X_n)/n$. then

$$P\left[\sqrt{n}\,(\bar{X}_n-\mu)/\sigma < x\right] \to \Phi(x)$$

This result is proved for the special case where the moment generating function exists in A106.

A89. TRANSFORMATIONS (CONTINUOUS VARIABLES) (Consequence)

Let $X = (X_1, \ldots, X_n)$ be a vector of continuous random variables with joint probability density

$$f_X(x_1, \ldots, x_n)$$

Let $Y = (Y_1, \ldots, Y_n)$ where $Y_j = g_j(X_1, \ldots, X_n)$ $j=1,2,\ldots,n$ be a $1-1$ function of X. That is, no two different X vectors produce the same Y vector. Let $K = K(X)$ be the matrix function whose i^{th} row, j^{th} column is

$$K_{ij}(X) = \frac{\partial g_j}{\partial x_i}(X) \qquad 1 \le i \le n, \quad 1 \le j \le n$$

Then Y has joint density

$$f_Y(y_1, \ldots, y_n) = \frac{f_X(x_1, \ldots, x_n)}{|\det(K)|}$$

with

$$\det(K) = \text{Determinant}$$

$$|\ \ | = \text{Absolute value}$$

$$y_j = g_j(x_1, \ldots, x_n)$$

The reader is referred to Hogg and Craig (1978) for further details, but an example might be helpful.

A90. Example

Let $X_1, X_2, \ldots, X_n$ be independent exponential random variables with common parameter λ.

$$f_X(x_1, \ldots, x_n) = \lambda^n \exp\left\{-\lambda(x_1 + \cdots + x_n)\right\} \qquad x_j > 0$$

Let

$$Y_1 = X_1$$

$$Y_2 = X_1 + X_2$$

$$Y_j = X_1 + \cdots + X_j$$

$$\vdots$$

$$Y_n = X_1 + \cdots + X_n$$

Note

$$X_1 = Y_1$$

$$X_2 = Y_2 - Y_1$$

$$X_3 = Y_3 - Y_2$$

$$\vdots$$

$$X_n = Y_n - Y_{n-1}$$

Hence, the value of the X's is uniquely determined by the Y's.

$$y_j = g_j(x_1, \ldots, x_n) = x_1 + \cdots + x_j$$

$$\frac{\partial g_j}{\partial x_i} = 1 \qquad i \leq j$$

$$= 0 \qquad i > j$$

$$K = \begin{bmatrix} 1 & 0 & 0 & \cdots & 0 \\ 1 & 1 & 0 & \cdots & 0 \\ 1 & 1 & 1 & 0 & 0 \\ \vdots & \vdots & \vdots & \vdots & \vdots \\ 1 & \cdots & \cdots & \cdots & 1 \end{bmatrix}$$

$$\det(K) = 1$$

$$f_Y(y_1, \ldots, y_n) = \lambda^n \exp\left\{-\lambda(x_1 + \cdots + x_n)\right\}$$
$$= \lambda^n \exp\left\{-\lambda y_n\right\}$$

Now the range of the y's is obtained from the range of x's as

$$0 < x_1 < x_1 + x_2 < x_1 + x_2 + x_3 \ldots$$

$$0 < y_1 < y_2 < \cdots < y_n < \infty.$$

CONVERGENCE

A91. Limit of a Sequence (Definition)

Let $A_1, A_2, \ldots, A_n, \ldots$ be a sequence of constants. We say that A_n converges to the constant A,

($A_n \rightarrow A$) if for every $\epsilon > 0$, there exists a number $N = N(\epsilon)$ such that whenever

$$n > N, \quad |A_n - A| < \epsilon.$$

In other words, you challenge me with a tiny number ϵ. I find a large N such that

$$|A_n - A| < \epsilon \text{ for all } n > N.$$

This can be done for every $\epsilon > 0$.

Example: $A_n = 1/n$ $A=0$

$N(\epsilon) = 1/\epsilon$

A92. Convergence in Probability (Definition)

Let $X_1, X_2, \ldots, X_n \ldots$ be a sequence of random variables. We say that X_n converges in probability to the constant C

$$X_n \xrightarrow{P} C$$

If for every $\epsilon > 0$

$$P\left(|X_n - C| > \epsilon\right) \rightarrow 0 \text{ as } n \rightarrow \infty$$

In other words, regardless of what small "challenge number" ϵ you provide, the probability that X_n is within ϵ of C goes to one.

A93. Convergence in Distribution (Definition)

Let $X_1, X_2, \ldots$ be a sequence of random variables with respective cumulative distributions

$$F_1(x), F_2(x), \ldots, F_n(x), \ldots$$

We say that

$$F_n \rightarrow F \text{ in distribution}$$

if

$$F_n(x) \rightarrow F(x) \qquad \text{at every continuity point of x.}$$

This is denoted by $F_n \xrightarrow{D} F$ or $X_n \xrightarrow{D} F$.

A94. Convergence in Distribution (Consequence)

Let $X_1, X_2, \ldots$ be a sequence of random variables with respective cumulative distributions $F_1(x), F_2(x), \ldots$ and respective Moment Generating Functions

$$M_1(t), M_2(t), \ldots$$

Suppose that

$$M_n(t) \rightarrow M(t)$$

in a neighborhood of t=0 and M(t) is the Moment Generating Function of F(x). Then $F_n \xrightarrow{D} F$.

The proof is beyond the intended scope of the book. Interested readers might refer to Fraser (1976, pages 248 and 558-560.)

Convergence in Probability (Consequence)

A95. (i) If $X_n \xrightarrow{P} x$

and $Y_n = cX_n$ c constant

Then $Y_n \xrightarrow{P} cx$

A96. (ii) If $X_n \xrightarrow{P} x$

and $Y_n \xrightarrow{P} 0$

then $X_n Y_n \xrightarrow{P} 0$

A97. (iii) If $X_n \xrightarrow{P} x$ and $x \neq 0$,

then if $Y_n = 1/X_n$

$Y_n \xrightarrow{P} (1/x)$

A98. (iv) If $X_n \xrightarrow{P} x$ and g is continuous at x

then $g(X_n) \xrightarrow{P} g(x)$

Proofs:

(i) If $c = 0$, then $Y_n = 0 = cx$ for all n and the result is immediate

If $c \neq 0$

$$P\left[|Y_n - cx| > \epsilon\right] = P\left[|X_n - x| > \frac{\epsilon}{|c|}\right] \to 0 \quad \text{since } X_n \xrightarrow{P} x$$

That is, $Y_n \xrightarrow{P} cx$

(ii) The event that $|X_n Y_n| < \epsilon$ contains the intersection of the events

$|X_n - x| < \epsilon$ (event A_n)

and $|Y_n| < \frac{\epsilon}{|x|+\epsilon}$ (event B_n)

(Event A_n implies that $|X_n| < |x| + \epsilon$ and hence A_n and B_n together imply $|X_n Y_n| < \epsilon$.).

$$\begin{aligned} P(A_n B_n) &= P(A_n) - P(A_n \bar{B}_n) \\ &\geq P(A_n) - P(\bar{B}_n) \end{aligned}$$

Now $P(A_n) \to 1$ since $X_n \xrightarrow{P} x$

and $P(\bar{B}_n) \to 0$ since $Y_n \xrightarrow{P} 0$.

Hence $P(A_n B_n) \to 1$.

$$P\left[|X_n Y_n| < \epsilon\right] \geq P\left(A_n B_n\right) \to 1 \text{ as } n \to \infty.$$

(iii) This is an important special case of (iv).

(iv) Given $\epsilon > 0$, there exists a $\delta > 0$ such that whenever $|y - x| < \delta$, $|g(y) - g(x)| < \epsilon$.

Above is the definition of continuity.

Therefore, the event that $|g(X_n) - g(x)| < \epsilon$ contains the event A_n, that $|X_n - x| < \delta$. But

$$P[A_n] = P\left[|X_n - x| < \delta\right] \to 1 \qquad \text{(Convergence in P)}$$

Convergence in Probability (Consequence)

Let $X_n \xrightarrow{P} x$ and $Y_n \xrightarrow{P} y$. Then

A99. (v) $X_n + Y_n \xrightarrow{P} x+y$

A100. (vi) $X_n - Y_n \xrightarrow{P} x-y$

A101. (vii) $X_n Y_n \xrightarrow{P} xy$

A102. (viii) $X_n/Y_n \xrightarrow{P} x/y$ if $y \neq 0$

Proofs:

(v) The event that $|X_n + Y_n - x - y| < \epsilon$ contains the event that both $|X_n - x| < \frac{\epsilon}{2}$ and $|Y_n - y| < \frac{\epsilon}{2}$.

$$P\left[|X_n - x| < \tfrac{\epsilon}{2}, |Y_n - y| < \tfrac{\epsilon}{2}\right] = P\left[|X_n - x| < \tfrac{\epsilon}{2}\right] - P\left[|X_n - x| < \tfrac{\epsilon}{2}, |Y_n - y| \geq \tfrac{\epsilon}{2}\right]$$

$$\geq P\left[|X_n - x| < \tfrac{\epsilon}{2}\right] - P\left[|Y_n - y| \geq \tfrac{\epsilon}{2}\right] \rightarrow 1 - 0 = 1 \text{ as } n \rightarrow \infty.$$

i.e., $P\left[|X_n + Y_n - x - y| < \epsilon\right] \rightarrow 1$

(vi) By (i), $-Y_n \xrightarrow{P} -y$. Apply (v) to get desired result.

(vii) $X_n Y_n - xy = X_n(Y_n - y) + (X_n - x)y$

Now by (ii), $X_n(Y_n - y) \xrightarrow{P} 0$

and by (i), $(X_n - x)y \xrightarrow{P} 0$

Hence, by (v) $X_n Y_n - xy \xrightarrow{P} 0$

(viii) By (iii) $\frac{1}{Y_n} \xrightarrow{P} \frac{1}{y}$. Results hold by (vii) above.

A103. Convergence in Probability (Consequence)

If $\frac{A_n}{B_n} \xrightarrow{P} 1$

$\frac{C_n}{D_n} \xrightarrow{P} 1$

with $A_n, B_n, C_n, D_n > 0$

then $\frac{A_n + C_n}{B_n + D_n} \xrightarrow{P} 1$

Proof: Let $\epsilon>0$, $\delta>0$. Then there exists $N_1>0$ and $N_2>0$,

$$n>N_1 \Rightarrow P\left[1-\epsilon < \left(\frac{A_n}{B_n}\right) < 1+\epsilon\right] > 1-\frac{\delta}{2}$$

$$n>N_2 \Rightarrow P\left[1-\epsilon < \left(\frac{C_n}{D_n}\right) < 1+\epsilon\right] > 1-\frac{\delta}{2}$$

$$n>\max(N_1, N_2) \Rightarrow P\left[B_n(1-\epsilon) < A_n < B_n(1+\epsilon)\right] > 1-\frac{\delta}{2}$$

$$P\left[D_n(1-\epsilon) < C_n < D_n(1+\epsilon)\right] > 1-\frac{\delta}{2}.$$

The event

$$1-\epsilon < \frac{A_n + C_n}{B_n + D_n} < 1 + \epsilon$$

includes the intersection of the events

$$B_n(1-\epsilon) < A_n < B_n(1+\epsilon)$$

with $D_n(1-\epsilon) < C_n < D_n(1+\epsilon)$ and hence

$$P\left[1-\epsilon < \frac{A_n+C_n}{B_n+D_n} < 1+\epsilon\right] > 1-\delta.$$

Since ϵ and δ are arbitrary, the desired result holds.

A104. Convergence in Distribution (Consequence)

Slutzky's Theorem

Let $X_1, X_2, \ldots$ be a sequence of random variables with cumulative distributions

$F_1, F_2, \ldots$, with $X_n \xrightarrow{D} F$.

Let Y_n be a sequence of random variables with $Y_n \xrightarrow{P} 0$.

Then if $Z_n = X_n + Y_n$, and if we denote the cumulative distribution of Z_n by G_n, then

$$Z_n \xrightarrow{D} F \qquad (G_n \xrightarrow{D} F)$$

Note: We shall prove the result under the mild restriction that F(x) has "isolated discontinuities." That is, at each point x_0 such that F has a jump at x_0, there exists an $h>0$ such that F is continuous in the intervals (x_0-h, x_0) and (x_0, x_0+h). Continuous distributions and discrete distributions over the integers have this property. [A discrete distribution over the rational numbers is pathological, and does not have this property.]

Proof: Let x be a continuity point of F and let

A_n be the event that $X_n \le x-\delta$

B_n be the event that $Y_n \le \delta$

C_n be the event that $X_n+Y_n \le x$.

Since C_n contains the intersection of A_n and B_n

$$\begin{aligned} G_n(x) = P(C_n) &\ge P(A_nB_n) \\ &\ge P(A_n) - P(A_n\bar{B}_n) \\ &\ge P(A_n) - P(\bar{B}_n) \end{aligned}$$

$$G_n(x) \ge F_n(x-\delta) - P(Y_n > \delta) \tag{1}$$

Similarly, if A_n^* is the event that $X_n > x+\delta$

B_n^* is the event that $Y_n > -\delta$

C_n^* is the event that $X_n + Y_n > x$

C_n^* contains the intersection of A_n^* and B_n^* and hence

$$1-G_n(x) \ge 1-F_n(x+\delta) - P(Y_n \le -\delta)$$

i.e.,

$$G_n(x) \le F_n(x+\delta) + P(Y_n \le -\delta) \tag{2}$$

Combining (1) and (2) we have

$$F_n(x-\delta) - P(Y_n>\delta) \le G_n(x) \le F_n(x+\delta) + P(Y_n \le -\delta). \tag{3}$$

Since discontinuities are isolated, we can restrict our attention to $\delta < h$, where F is continuous in the interval $(x-h, x+h)$.

In (3), as $n\to\infty$ $\quad F_n(x+\delta) \to F(x+\delta)$

$$F_n(x-\delta) \to F(x-\delta)$$

by convergence in distribution.

Also, $\quad P(Y_n>\delta)$ and $P(Y_n\le -\delta)\to 0$

since $\quad Y_n \xrightarrow{P} 0.$

Hence: $\quad \lim_{n\to\infty}\left\{F_n(x-\delta) - P(Y_n>\delta)\right\} = F(x-\delta)$

and $\quad \lim_{n\to\infty}\left\{F_n(x+\delta) + P(Y_n \le -\delta\right\} = F(x+\delta).$

Let $\epsilon>0$ be arbitrary. Then there exists $N_1 = N_1(\epsilon,\delta)$ and $N_2 = N_2(\epsilon,\delta)$ such that whenever $n>N_1$

$$G_n(x) \ge F_n(x-\delta) - P(Y_n>\delta) > F(x-\delta) - \epsilon$$

and whenever $n>N_2$

$$G_n(x) \le F_n(x+\delta) + P(Y_n \le -\delta) < F(x+\delta) + \epsilon.$$

That is, whenever $n > \text{Max}(N_1, N_2)$

$$F(x-\delta) - \epsilon < G_n(x) < F(x+\delta) + \epsilon. \tag{4}$$

Finally, from the continuity of F at x, there exists δ_0 such that

$|F(x) - F(y)| \le \epsilon$ $\quad$ whenever

$|x-y| < \delta_0$.

From (4), we have whenever

$$n > \text{Max}\left\{N_1(\epsilon, \delta_0), N_2(\epsilon, \delta_0)\right\}$$

$$F(x) - 2\epsilon < G_n(x) < F(x) + 2\epsilon.$$

Since ϵ is arbitrary, we conclude that

$$G_n(x) \to F(x) \qquad \text{as } n\to\infty.$$

This completes the proof.

A105. Slutzky's Theorem for Products (Consequence)

Let $X_n \xrightarrow{D} F$ and $Y_n \xrightarrow{P} 1$

then $Z_n = X_n Y_n \xrightarrow{D} F$

Note: We shall prove the result under the same isolated discontinuity assumption as the previous result.

Proof: It is clear that

$$X_n Y_n = X_n + X_n(Y_n\text{-}1)$$

If we can show

$$X_n(Y_n\text{-}1) \xrightarrow{P} 0$$

the desired result is immediate from the previous result.

Suppose we are challenged with two small number, δ and ϵ.

First, since F is a proper distribution we can find a real number B such that both B and -B are continuity points of F and

$$F(B) - F(-B) > 1\text{-}\delta$$

Let A_n be the event that $-B < X_n \leq B$ and B_n be the event that $|Y_n\text{-}1| < \epsilon/B$.

The event that $|X_n(Y_n\text{-}1)| < \epsilon$ contains the intersection of A_n and B_n.

$$\begin{aligned} P(A_n B_n) &= P(A_n) - P(A_n \bar{B}_n) \\ &\geq P(A_n) - P(\bar{B}_n) \\ &\geq F_n(B) - F_n(-B) - P(\bar{B}_n) \\ &\rightarrow F(B) - F(-B) \quad \text{as } n \rightarrow \infty \\ &> 1\text{-}\delta. \end{aligned}$$

i.e., since we can make δ as close to zero as we wish, and since $|X_n(Y_n\text{-}1)| < \epsilon$ whenever $A_n B_n$ holds,

$$|X_n(Y_n\text{-}1)| \xrightarrow{P} 0.$$

This completes the proof.

A106. Central Limit Theorem for Independent, Identically Distributed Random Variables

Let $X_1, X_2, \ldots, X_n \cdots$ be independent, identically distributed random variables with mean μ, variance σ^2, and moment generating function $M_X(t)$.

Then $Z_n = \dfrac{n^{\frac{1}{2}}(\bar{X}_n - \mu)}{\sigma} \xrightarrow{D} N(0,1)$ where $\bar{X}_n = \dfrac{(X_1 + \cdots + X_n)}{n}$ and N(0,1) is the standard normal distribution.

Proof. It is seen from **A56 and A40** that Z_n has moment generating function

$$M_{Z_n}(\theta) = \left[M_X\left(\frac{\theta}{\sigma\sqrt{n}}\right)\right]^n \exp\left[\frac{-\sqrt{n}\mu\theta}{\sigma}\right].$$

We need to show (See **A94 and A85**) that

$$M_{Z_n}(\theta) \to e^{\theta^2/2} \qquad \text{in a neighborhood of } \theta = 0.$$

That is, we must show

$$K_n(\theta) = \log M_{Z_n}(\theta) \to \frac{\theta^2}{2} \qquad \text{in a neighborhood of } \theta = 0. \tag{0}$$

$$K_n(\theta) = n \log M_X\left(\frac{\theta}{\sigma\sqrt{n}}\right) - \frac{\sqrt{n}\mu\theta}{\sigma} \tag{1}$$

By Taylor's Theorem, there exists θ^*: $|\theta^*|<|\theta|$

$$K_n(\theta) = K_n(0) + \theta K_n'(0) + \frac{\theta^2}{2}K_n''(0) + \frac{\theta^3}{6}K_n'''(\theta^*). \tag{2}$$

From (1), and the fact that $M_X(0) = E\left(e^{0X_n}\right) = 1$, we see that $K_n(0) = 0$

$$K_n'(\theta) = \frac{\sqrt{n}}{\sigma}\,\frac{M_X'\left\{\theta/(\sigma\sqrt{n})\right\}}{M_X\left\{\theta/(\sigma\sqrt{n})\right\}} - \frac{\sqrt{n}\mu}{\sigma} \tag{3}$$

$$K_n''(\theta) = \frac{1}{\sigma^2}\left[\frac{M_X''\{\theta/(\sigma\sqrt{n})\}}{M_X\{\theta/(\sigma\sqrt{n})\}} - \frac{\left[M_X'\{\theta/(\sigma\sqrt{n})\}\right]^2}{\left[M_X\{\theta/(\sigma\sqrt{n})\}\right]^2}\right] \tag{4}$$

$$K_n'''(\theta) = \frac{1}{\sqrt{n}\sigma^3}\left[\frac{M_X'''\{\theta/(\sigma\sqrt{n})\}}{M_X\{\theta/(\sigma\sqrt{n})\}} - \frac{3M_X''\{\theta/(\sigma\sqrt{n})\}M_X'\{\theta/(\sigma\sqrt{n})\}}{\left[M_X\{\theta/(\sigma\sqrt{n})\}\right]^2} + \frac{2\left[M_X'\{\theta/(\sigma\sqrt{n})\}\right]^3}{\left[M_X\{\theta/(\sigma\sqrt{n})\}\right]^3}\right] \tag{5}$$

$$K_n(0) = 0 \tag{6}$$

$$K_n'(0) = \frac{\sqrt{n}}{\sigma}\frac{M_X'(0)}{M_X(0)} - \frac{\sqrt{n}}{\sigma}\mu = 0 \tag{7}$$

$$K_n''(0) = \frac{1}{\sigma^2}\left[E(X_j^2) - \mu^2\right] = \frac{\sigma^2}{\sigma^2} = 1 \tag{8}$$

$K_n'''(\theta^*) \rightarrow 0$ as shown below. (9)

Let

$$L_n(y) = \frac{M_X'''(y)}{M_X(y)} - \frac{3M_X''(y)M_X'(y)}{\left[M_X(y)\right]^2} + \frac{2\left[M_X'(y)\right]^3}{\left[M_X(y)\right]^3}.$$

Now

$$K_n'''(\theta^*) = \frac{1}{\sqrt{n}\sigma^3}L_n\{\theta^*/(\sigma\sqrt{n})\}$$

and $L_n(y) \rightarrow E(X_j^3) - 3\mu E(X_j^2) + 2\mu^3$ as $y \rightarrow 0$, a finite quantity. Hence

$$\lim_{n\rightarrow\infty} K_n'''(\theta^*) = \lim_{n\rightarrow\infty}\left(\frac{1}{\sqrt{n}\sigma^3}\right) \lim_{n\rightarrow\infty} L_n\{\theta^*/(\sigma\sqrt{n})\} = 0. \tag{10}$$

From (2), (6), (7), (8) and (10) we have

$$K_n(\theta) \rightarrow \theta^2/2 \quad \text{as } n \rightarrow \infty.$$

This completes the proof, as the requirement of equation (0) has been met.

A107. A Central Limit Theorem for Sums of Bernoulli Random Variables

Let X_j, $j = 1, 2, \ldots, n$ be independent Bernoulli Random Variables (i.e., Binomial with sample size 1) with mass function

$$\begin{aligned} f_j(x) &= 1 - p_j & x &= 0 \\ &= p_j & x &= 1 \\ &= 0 & &\text{elsewhere.} \end{aligned}$$

Let b_j, $j = 1, 2, \ldots$ be constants and

$$S_n = \sum_{j=1}^{n} b_j X_j$$

$$M_n = \sum_{j=1}^{n} b_j p_j$$

$$V_n^2 = \sum_{j=1}^{n} b_j^2 p_j (1 - p_j)$$

and
$$Z_n = \frac{S_n - M_n}{V_n}$$

Without loss of generality in what follows, the b_j, p_j (and hence X_j) may be functions of n. We dropped the subscript n for ease of notation.

A107-1 Condition 1:

If $V_n \to \infty$

and

$$\frac{\sum_{j=1}^{n} |b_j|^3}{V_n^3} \to 0 \text{ as } n \to \infty.$$

then

$$Z_n \xrightarrow{D} N(0,1) \quad \text{(Standard Normal).}$$

A107-2 Condition 2:

If the b_j and p_j are bounded:

$$p_j < p_0 < 1 \text{ and } |b_j| < B$$

and

$$V_n \to \infty$$

and if

$$\frac{\sum_{j=1}^{n} |b_j|^3 p_j}{V_n^3} \to 0 \quad \text{as } n \to \infty$$

then

$$Z_n \xrightarrow{D} N(0,1).$$

This is designed to cover cases where $p_j \to 0$.

Proof. Let

$$K_n(\theta) = \log E\left(e^{\theta Z_n}\right) \tag{0}$$

the log of the moment generating function of Z_n.

It is readily seen by independence that

$$K_n(\theta) = \sum_{j=1}^{n} \left\{ \log \left[(1-p_j) + p_j e^{b_j\theta/V_n} \right] - \frac{b_j p_j \theta}{V_n} \right\} \tag{1}$$

To prove normality, we need to show that

$$K_n(\theta) \to \frac{\theta^2}{2} \quad \text{as } n \to \infty$$

in a neighborhood of $\theta = 0$.

By Taylor's Theorem, there exists a θ^* such that $|\theta^*| \le |\theta|$ with

$$K_n(\theta) = K_n(0) + \theta K_n'(0) + \frac{\theta^2}{2} K_n''(0) + \frac{\theta^3}{6} K_n'''(\theta^*). \tag{2}$$

$$K_n'(\theta) = \sum_{j=1}^{n} \frac{b_j p_j}{V_n} \left\{ \frac{1}{(1-p_j)e^{-b_j\theta/V_n} + p_j} - 1 \right\}. \tag{3}$$

$$K_n''(\theta) = \sum_{j=1}^{n} \frac{b_j^2 p_j(1-p_j)}{V_n^2} \frac{e^{-b_j\theta/V_n}}{\left\{(1-p_j)e^{-b_j\theta/V_n} + p_j\right\}^2}. \tag{4}$$

$$K_n'''(\theta) = 2\sum_{j=1}^{n} \frac{b_j^3 p_j(1-p_j)^2 e^{-2b_j\theta/V_n}}{V_n^3\left\{(1-p_j)e^{-b_j\theta/V_n} + p_j\right\}^3} - \sum_{j=1}^{n} \frac{b_j^3 p_j(1-p_j)e^{-b_j\theta/V_n}}{V_n^3\left\{(1-p_j)e^{-b_j\theta/V_n} + p_j\right\}^2}. \tag{5}$$

Clearly, $K_n(0) = 0$ (Substitute $\theta = 0$ in (1)).

By substituting $\theta = 0$ in (3), we see that

$$\begin{aligned}(1 - p_j)e^{-b_j\theta/V_n} + p_j &= (1 - p_j)e^0 + p_j \\ &= 1.\end{aligned}$$

Hence $\quad K_n'(0) = 0.$

Similarly, from (4),

$$K_n''(0) = \sum_{j=1}^{n} \frac{b_j^2 p_j(1 - p_j)}{V_n^2} = \frac{V_n^2}{V_n^2} = 1.$$

To prove Condition 1, consider in (5)

$$\frac{p_j}{(1 - p_j)e^{-b_j\theta/V_n} + p_j} \leq 1,$$

and
$$\frac{(1 - p_j)e^{-b_j\theta/V_n}}{(1 - p_j)e^{-b_j\theta/V_n} + p_j} \leq 1.$$

Hence

$$|K_n'''(\theta)| < 3\,\frac{\Sigma|b_j|^3}{V_n^3} \tag{6}$$

Since the right hand side of (6) converges to zero, convergence to zero of $K_n'''(\theta)$ is assured.

From (2)

$$K_n(\theta) \rightarrow \frac{\theta^2}{2}$$

and hence

$$E\left(e^{\theta Z_n}\right) \rightarrow e^{\theta^2/2} \qquad n\rightarrow\infty.$$

That is from A94,

$Z_n \xrightarrow{D} N(0,1)$ under condition 1.

For Condition 2, note that since $V_n \rightarrow \infty$ there exists for given $V_0 > 0$, a number N such that whenever

$$n > N, \qquad V_n > V_0.$$

Now working with (5) we see

$$\frac{1}{(1 - p_j)e^{-b_j\theta/V_n} + p_j} \leq \frac{1}{(1 - p_j)e^{-b_j\theta/V_n}} \leq \frac{e^{|b_j\theta|/V_n}}{1 - p_j} \leq \frac{e^{|B\theta|/V_0}}{1 - p_0} \qquad n > N,$$

also

$$\frac{(1 - p_j)e^{-b_j\theta/V_n}}{(1 - p_j)e^{-b_j\theta/V_n} + p_j} \leq 1.$$

Hence for n > N, Condition 2 and (5) yield

$$|K_n'''(\theta)| < \frac{3e^{|B\theta|/V_0}}{1 - p_0} \left\{ \frac{\sum_{j=1}^{n} |b_j|^3 p_j}{V_n^3} \right\} \qquad \text{for } n > N$$

$$\rightarrow 0.$$

Hence $\quad K_n(\theta) \rightarrow \frac{\theta^2}{2}$

and hence $\quad E\left(e^{\theta Z_n}\right) \rightarrow e^{\theta^2/2},$

and hence from **A94**,

$$Z_n \xrightarrow{D} N(0,1) \text{ under Condition 2.}$$

A107-EX Example:

$$p_j = p_j(n) = \frac{1}{\sqrt{n}}$$

$$b_j = 1$$

$$V_n^2 = n\left(\frac{1}{\sqrt{n}}\right)\left(1 - \frac{1}{\sqrt{n}}\right) = \sqrt{n} - 1$$

$$b_j^3 = 1 \text{ and } \Sigma b_j^3 = n$$

$$\frac{\Sigma b_j^3}{V_n^3} = \frac{n}{\left\{\sqrt{n}-1\right\}^{\frac{3}{2}}} \sim n^{\frac{1}{4}} \quad \text{(Condition 1 fails, since this does not go to zero).}$$

$$\frac{\Sigma b_j^3 p_j}{V_n^3} = \frac{\sqrt{n}}{\left\{\sqrt{n}-1\right\}^{\frac{3}{2}}} \to 0 \quad \text{(Condition 2 succeeds).}$$

A108 Asymptotic Normality of a Difference

Suppose X_n and Y_n are independent with

$$\frac{X_n - \mu_n}{\sigma_n} \xrightarrow{D} N(0, 1)$$

$$\frac{Y_n - \nu_n}{\lambda_n} \xrightarrow{D} N(0, 1)$$

$$\frac{\sigma_n}{\lambda_n} \to c$$

where μ_n, ν_n, σ_n, λ_n are constants.

Then
$$\frac{(X_n-Y_n) - (\mu_n-\nu_n)}{\sqrt{\sigma_n^2 + \lambda_n^2}} \xrightarrow{D} N(0, 1)$$

Proof:

$$\frac{X_n-\mu_n}{\sqrt{\sigma_n^2 + \lambda_n^2}} = \frac{X_n- \mu_n}{\sigma_n\sqrt{\left(1 + \frac{\lambda_n^2}{\sigma_n^2}\right)}}.$$

Now since $\frac{\lambda_n^2}{\sigma_n^2} \to c^{-2}$,

Slutzky's Multiplicative Theorem A105 implies

$$\frac{X_n - \mu_n}{\sqrt{\sigma_n^2 + \lambda_n^2}} \text{ and } \frac{X_n - \mu_n}{\sigma_n \sqrt{1 + c^{-2}}}$$

have the same asymptotic distribution. That is

$$\frac{X_n - \mu_n}{\sqrt{\sigma_n^2 + \lambda_n^2}} \xrightarrow{D} N\left(0, \frac{1}{1+c^{-2}}\right).$$

Similarly,

$$\frac{Y_n - \nu_n}{\sqrt{\sigma_n^2 + \lambda_n^2}} = \frac{Y_n - \nu_n}{\lambda_n \sqrt{1 + \frac{\sigma_n^2}{\lambda_n^2}}} \xrightarrow{D} N\left(0, \frac{1}{1+c^2}\right)$$

From A87,

$$\frac{(X_n - Y_n) - (\mu_n - \nu_n)}{\sqrt{\sigma_n^2 + \lambda_n^2}} \xrightarrow{D} N\left(0, \frac{1}{1+c^2} + \frac{1}{1+c^{-2}}\right)$$

But

$$\frac{1}{1+c^2} + \frac{1}{1+c^{-2}} = \frac{1}{1+c^2} + \frac{c^2}{1+c^2} = 1$$

Therefore

$$\frac{(X_n - Y_n) - (\mu_n - \nu_n)}{\sqrt{\sigma_n^2 + \lambda_n^2}} \xrightarrow{D} N(0, 1)$$

A109. Asymptotic Normality of a Difference

If in addition to the conditions of **A108**, we have consistent estimators

$$\frac{\hat{\sigma}_n}{\sigma_n} \xrightarrow{P} 1$$

$$\frac{\hat{\lambda}_n}{\lambda_n} \xrightarrow{P} 1$$

Then

$$\frac{(X_n - Y_n) - (\mu_n - \nu_n)}{\sqrt{\hat{\sigma}_n^2 + \hat{\lambda}_n^2}} \xrightarrow{D} N(0, 1)$$

Proof: By A98,

$$\frac{\hat{\sigma}_n^2}{\sigma_n^2} \xrightarrow{P} 1$$

$$\frac{\hat{\lambda}_n^2}{\lambda_n^2} \xrightarrow{P} 1.$$

Hence by A103,

$$\frac{\hat{\sigma}_n^2 + \hat{\lambda}_n^2}{\sigma_n^2 + \lambda_n^2} \xrightarrow{P} 1.$$

Again using A98, this yields

$$\frac{\sqrt{\hat{\sigma}_n^2 + \hat{\lambda}_n^2}}{\sqrt{\sigma_n^2 + \lambda_n^2}} \xrightarrow{P} 1.$$

Finally, from A108 snd Slutsky's Theorem (Products), A105, the desired result holds.

STATISTICAL INFERENCE

A110 Estimator of a Parameter (Definition)

A random variable, whose observed value will estimate a parameter.

Example: The sample mean is an estimator of the population mean.

If the parameter is θ, then the estimator is denoted by $\hat{\theta}$

A111 Unbiased Estimator (Definition)

$\hat{\theta}$ is "unbiased" for θ if $E(\hat{\theta}) = \theta$

A112 Consistent Estimator(s) (Definition)

Let $\hat{\theta}_1, \hat{\theta}_2, \ldots$ be a sequence of estimators of θ. $\hat{\theta}_n$ is "consistent" for θ if

$$\hat{\theta}_n \xrightarrow{P} \theta.$$

(More formally, this is called "weakly consistent".)

A113 Maximum Likelihood Estimator

$\hat{\theta}$ is said to be the Maximum Likelihood Estimator of θ if the probability of the observed sample (discrete case) or joint density of the observed sample (continuous case) is maximized at $\theta = \hat{\theta}$.

This is a technique to obtain estimators of θ. In many applications, they are consistent, asymptotically normal, with optimal asymptotic variance.

We shall not make use of these estimators directly, but we include the definition for the sake of completeness.

A114 Confidence Interval (Definition)

Consider two estimators $\hat{\theta}_L < \hat{\theta}_U$ such that the pre-experiment probability

$$P\left[\hat{\theta}_L < \theta < \hat{\theta}_U\right] = (1 - \alpha).$$

We say that

$$\left(\hat{\theta}_L, \hat{\theta}_U\right)$$

form a 100(1-α)% confidence interval for θ.

After the data has been collected, probability no longer applies. $\hat{\theta}_L$, θ, and $\hat{\theta}_U$ are simply three numbers. We do have 100(1-α)% confidence in our procedure to capture the true θ. [The analogy is the following. Before playing a key ball game, Team A was believed to have a 90% chance of defeating team B. You might consider betting on the outcome. Even if you did not know the true result, but you did know that the game was over, you would not bet on the game.]

HYPOTHESIS TESTING (*P*-values)

A115 Null Hypothesis (Definition)

A statement corresponding to an unsuccessful outcome of an experiment or study. This is generally expressed in terms of parameters. The objective of the study will be achieved if we can reject the null hypothesis in favor of the alternate hypothesis below. We denote this by H_0.

A116 Alternate Hypothesis (Definition)

A statement corresponding to a successful outcome of an experiment or study. We denote this by H_A.

A117 Example (i):

Suppose you wish to determine which of two therapies is better in terms of five year survival. Since it is inconceivable that the five year survival under each therapy is exactly equal, the goal of the study is to find out which is better. The null hypothesis would be that the five year survival of each therapy is exactly the same. The alternative hypothesis is that there is a difference.

$$H_0 : P_5 = Q_5 \quad \text{versus} \quad H_A : P_5 \neq Q_5$$

with P_5 and Q_5 the five year survival under treatment A and treatment B respectively. If you can conclude beyond a reasonable doubt that one of the treatments is superior to the other (reject H_0), your research question will have been answered. If you fail to reject H_0, you <u>do not</u> conclude that the treatments are equal in terms of five year survival, but rather, that the data are <u>inconclusive</u>.

This is called a <u>two tailed test</u>. The burden of evidence is always placed on rejecting H_0 in favor of H_A.

A118 Example (ii):

Suppose that you wish to determine if the addition of a drug to a "standard" treatment improves five year survival, over the standard treatment alone. You wish to place the burden of proof on showing that the addition of the drug has efficacy. In this situation, we have

$$H_0 : P_5 \leq Q_5 \quad \text{versus} \quad H_A : P_5 > Q_5$$

In such situations, if you cannot demonstrate beyond a reasonable doubt that P_5, the five year survival of the "experimental" therapy (standard plus drug) is greater than Q_5, the five year survival of the "control" therapy (standard alone), then the drug is considered unproven in terms of efficacy, over and above the standard.

This is called a <u>one tailed test</u>. The burden of proof is to show a difference in a specified direction.

Note: Some authors will write the one-tailed test as

$$H_0 : P_5 = Q_5 \text{ (instead of } H_0 : P_5 \leq Q_5) \quad \text{versus} \quad H_A : P_5 > Q_5$$

This is the most difficult situation among the candidates, where the more general H_0 is true, to distinguish H_0 from H_A. For example, it is harder to distinguish between hypotheses for situation (A) below than situation (B):

Situation (A): $P_5 = Q_5 = .20$ versus $P_5 = .20 \ Q_5 = .10$

Situation (B): $P_5 = .10 \ Q_5 = .20$ versus $P_5 = .20 \ Q_5 = .10$

A119 <u>Test Statistic</u> (Definition)

A quantity, calculated from the data, upon which the hypothesis test will be based. (The test statistic is simply the value of a random variable.)

A120 <u>P-Value</u> (Definition)

The maximum probability that in a replication of the study where the <u>null hypothesis is true</u>, that the test statistic would be at <u>least as "extreme"</u> as the observed test statistic (from the actual study.)

A121 <u>Two-Tailed Example</u> :

Suppose you wanted to determine which of two candidates is preferred. We might sample N = 400 individuals and assume that p = true proportion favoring A and 1-p = true proportion favoring B. Our hypotheses are

$$H_0 : p = .50 \quad \text{versus} \quad H_A ; p \neq .50$$

The test statistic generally used is

$$Z = 2\sqrt{n}(\hat{p} - .50)$$

where $\hat{p}$ is the fraction of the sample favoring A.

"Extreme" values for Z simply means large absolute values, since the larger $|Z|$ is, the stronger the evidence against H_0.

Under H_0, Z has an approximate standard normal distribution (see **A107**).

If for example, $\hat{p} = \frac{176}{400} = .440,$

$Z = -2.40.$

The p-value, as obtained from Figure 7, is p = .018. This provides strong evidence against H_0, and in favor of Candidate B.

A122 <u>One-Tailed Example:</u>

Via a randomized trial, a drug company wishes to show that their experimental agent combination can place a higher proportion of relapsed acute lymphocytic leukemia patients into remission than can the standard agent combination. If P_E and P_S are the experimental and standard remission rates respectively, we wish to test

$$H_0 : P_E \leq P_S \quad \text{versus} \quad H_A : P_E > P_S.$$

The test statistic used will be

$$Z = \frac{\hat{P}_E - \hat{P}_S}{\sqrt{\left\{\frac{\hat{P}_E(1-\hat{P}_E)}{N_E} + \frac{\hat{P}_S(1-\hat{P}_S)}{N_S}\right\}}}$$

where $\hat{P}_E$ and $\hat{P}_S$ are the fraction of patients achieving a remission on the experimental and standard agents respectively, and N_E and N_S are the corresponding sample sizes.

It is readily shown from results taken in our Appendix A107, A108, and A109, that if $P_E = P_S$, the hardest case in H_0 to distinguish from H_A, then Z is asymptotically standard normal.

Suppose that the observed value of Z is

$$Z = 0.37.$$

From Figure 6, this yields a p-value of P = 0.36. This value is certainly in the reasonable doubt range, and hence, we cannot reject H_0 in favor of H_A.

The study should be viewed as inconclusive as far as whether or not the experimental combination is superior.

A123 Standard Reasonable Doubt Thresholds:

The most widely used standard of doubt is a p-value of P = .05. In many fields, values below .05 are considered to be conclusive while values above are considered inconclusive.

Other than standardization, there is no logical basis for the 5% figure.

A124 Planning a Study (Sample Size Determination)

In planning a study, there are several ingredients needed in order to evaluate the sample size.

These include
- Null Hypothesis
- Alternative Hypothesis
- Test Statistic

A125
- "Type I Error." (α) Threshold p-value where you consider the dividing line between reasonable doubt and beyond reasonable doubt lies.) (This is usually denoted by α.)

A126 - "Planning Parameters." Under the alternate hypothesis, specify the parameters so that distributional properties of the test statistic can be evaluated. Generally, this involves specifying the smallest detectable difference of interest to the investigators, and other quantities such as accrual rate, "nuisance" parameters, and minimum follow-up time.

A127 - "Type II Error."(β) Specify the probability of failing to reject the null hypothesis, when the planning parameters represent the true target population conditions. (This is usually denoted by β.)

A128 - "Power" = 1 - Type II Error = probability of rejecting the null hypothesis when the planning parameters represent the true target population conditions. (This is usually denote by $\prod$.)

A129. The most common situation is the following: We shall show this as one-sided.

$$H_0\text{: } \theta = \theta_0 \text{ (or } H_0 : \theta \leq \theta_0) \qquad \text{versus} \qquad H_A : \theta > \theta_0$$

$$\text{Test Statistic: } Z = \frac{\hat{\theta} - \theta_0}{\text{SE}}$$

with SE = "Standard Error" of $\hat{\theta}$, (estimated standard deviation of $\hat{\theta}$), calculated from the data and

$Z \sim N(0,1)$ approximately, when H_0 is true.

To plan a study, enough information must be supplied to obtain an approximate distribution of Z under H_A.

This may involve specification of nuisance parameters.

For example, suppose that the planner of the acute lymphocytic leukemia study had come to you prior to conducting the study saying (see Chapter 2, Section 2.1.1)

"The study needs to be sensitive to a 10% difference. Type I Error should be $\alpha =$

.05 and Type II Error should be β = .20. I want equal sample sizes in each group."

$$H_0 : P_E - P_S = 0 \quad \text{versus} \quad H_A : P_E - P_S = .10$$

Test Statistic:

$$Z = \frac{\hat{P}_E - \hat{P}_S}{\sqrt{\left\{\frac{\hat{P}_E(1-\hat{P}_E)}{N_E} + \frac{\hat{P}_S(1-\hat{P}_S)}{N_S}\right\}}}$$

where $N = N_E + N_S$ = Total Sample Size

N_E = Number assigned to Experimental Therapy

N_S = Number assigned to Standard Therapy.

Z is approximately standard normal under H_0, but the approximate distribution of Z under H_A depends heavily on the actual values of P_E and P_S, not just the difference. The planner needs to provide values for both P_E and P_S under H_A to compute the sample size.

"Jumping ahead" somewhat, the required sample size in each group is: (See formal derivation in A132).

$$N_E = N_S = 617.5\left\{P_E(1-P_E) + P_S(1-P_S)\right\}$$

$= 56 \quad P_S = 0, P_E = .1$ (lowest possible value)

$= 306 \quad P_S = .45, P_E = .55$ (highest possible value)

It is much easier to distinguish 0 from 10% than it is to distinguish 45% from 55%.

A130 Sample Size Determination

The following derivation has not been developed in any text, yet is the basic background to nearly every sample size derivation. The ideas will look peculiar at first glance, but will make perfect sense once some examples are considered.

Consider the hypothesis:

$$H_0 : \theta = \theta_0 \quad \text{versus} \quad H_A : \theta = \theta_1 > \theta_0.$$

Let us set a Type I Error α and Power (1-β) (Type II Error β). Suppose that $\alpha + \beta < 1$.

Let us assume that we have statistics $\hat{\theta}$ and SE such that SE > 0,

$$\text{(a)} \quad P\left[\frac{\hat{\theta} - \theta_0}{SE} > Z_\alpha\right] \simeq \alpha \text{ under } H_0$$

and

$$\text{(b)} \quad P\left[\frac{\hat{\theta} - \theta_1}{SE} - \frac{(Z_\alpha + Z_\beta)(SE - S)}{SE} > - Z_\beta\right] \simeq 1 - \beta \text{ under } H_A,$$

with S, a function of the parameters of the distribution under H_A satisfying the implicit sample size equation:

$$S = \frac{\theta_1 - \theta_0}{Z_\alpha + Z_\beta} \qquad \text{(1). [KEY EQUATION]}$$

(Z_α and Z_β are generally the upper $(100\alpha)\%$ and $(100\beta)\%$ points of the standard normal distribution, but this derivation holds in general.)

Then

$$P\left[\frac{\hat{\theta} - \theta_0}{SE} > Z_\alpha\right] \simeq 1-\beta \text{ under } H_A.$$

That is, if S is given as per the (1) [key equation], then the rejection region

$$\hat{\theta} > \theta_0 + Z_\alpha SE$$

has approximate Type I Error α and Power 1 - β.

Proof:

This is simply a straight forward substitution for S in (b):

$$(1\text{-}\beta) \simeq P\left[\frac{\hat{\theta} - \theta_1}{SE} - \frac{(Z_\alpha + Z_\beta)(SE - S)}{SE} > -Z_\beta\right] \qquad \text{(under } H_A)$$

$$= P\left[\frac{\hat{\theta} - \theta_1 + (Z_\alpha + Z_\beta)S}{SE} - (Z_\alpha + Z_\beta) > -Z_\beta\right]$$

$$= P\left[\frac{\hat{\theta} - \theta_1 + (\theta_1 - \theta_0)}{SE} > Z_\alpha\right] \qquad (Z_\alpha + Z_\beta)S = \theta_1 - \theta_0$$

$$= P\left[\frac{\hat{\theta} - \theta_0}{SE} > Z_\alpha\right] \qquad \text{(under } H_A)$$

That is, the Type I and Power requirements are approximately met when equation (1) holds.

Note: S is the asymptotic standard deviation of the statistic under H_A, and may contain nuisance parameters. [SE usually has the same form as S, except population values under H_A (from S) are replaced by consistent estimators to obtain SE.]

A131 Extension to the two-sided test

For the two-sided test, we can replace α by $\alpha/2$ can utilize the equation

$$S = \frac{|\theta_1 - \theta_0|}{Z_{\alpha/2} + Z_\beta}$$

This implies two calculations, one for each alternative

$$H_A : \theta = \theta_1 = \theta_0 + \Delta \quad (\Delta > 0) \quad \text{and} \quad H_A : \theta = \theta_1 = \theta_0 - \Delta \quad (\Delta > 0)$$

The larger resulting sample size would be used.

A132 Example 1: Two Sample Independent Binomial with Equal Sample Sizes

The following notation will be used:

	Treatment 1	Treatment 2
Failure Rate	Q	T
Sample Size	N	N
Failures in Sample	F	G
Estimated Failure Rate	$\hat{Q} = F/N$	$\hat{T} = G/N$

$\theta = Q - T$

$H_0 : \theta = 0$

$H_A : \theta = \theta_1 > 0$

$\hat{\theta} = \hat{Q} - \hat{T}$

$$SE = \sqrt{\frac{\hat{Q}(1-\hat{Q})}{N} + \frac{\hat{T}(1-\hat{T})}{N}}$$

$$S = \sqrt{\frac{Q(1-Q)}{N} + \frac{T(1-T)}{N}}$$

For large N, we know

(i) $\frac{\hat{\theta} - 0}{SE} \rightarrow N(0,1)$ under H_0

(ii) $\frac{S}{SE} \xrightarrow{P} 1$ under H_A

(iii) $\frac{\hat{\theta} - \theta_1}{SE} \rightarrow N(0,1)$ under H_A

The approximation (a) of **A130** follows from (i), while from (ii), (iii) and Slutsky's theorem (**A104**), we have the approximation (b) of **A130**.

To obtain the sample size, we use

$$S = \frac{\theta_1 - \theta_0}{Z_\alpha + Z_\beta}.$$

Squaring both sides yields

$$\frac{Q(1\text{-}Q)}{N} + \frac{T(1\text{-}T)}{N} = \frac{(\theta_1 - \theta_0)^2}{(Z_\alpha + Z_\beta)^2} = \frac{(Q\text{-}T)^2}{(Z_\alpha + Z_\beta)^2}$$

That is, <u>each</u> sample size must be

A133 $$N = \frac{\left[Q(1\text{-}Q) + T(1\text{-}T)\right](Z_\alpha + Z_\beta)^2}{(Q\text{-}T)^2}$$

The two-tailed version of this formula appears in Pocock 1983, page 125.

A134 Example 2:

Let $Q = .7$ $T = .5$ in example 1, with $\alpha = .05$ and $\beta = .20$ (80% power), then

$$N = \frac{\left[.21 + .25\right](1.645 + .84)^2}{(.2)^2} = 71 \qquad \text{(each treatment)}$$

How good are these approximations? The exact binomial probability that the left hand term in assumption (a) exceeds 1.645 is 5.2% under H_0 (common $Q = T = .7$), while the exact binomial probability that the left hand term in assumption (b) exceeds -.84 is exactly 79.5% under H_A. These are very close to the asymptotic values of 5% and 80% respectively. For an exact approach to the two sample binomial problem see Suissa and Shuster (1985).

In the binomial example, we used a standard error valid under H_0 and H_A. We did not pool the proportions in the calculation.

A135 Summary of Sufficient Conditions to Apply the Sample Size Methodology

(1)	$\frac{(\hat{\theta} - \theta)}{SE}$	is asymptotically normal under H_0, $\theta = \theta_0$.
(2)	$\frac{(\hat{\theta} - \theta)}{SE}$	is asymptotically normal under H_A, $\theta = \theta_1$.
(3)	$\frac{S}{SE} \xrightarrow{P} 1$	under H_A.
(4)	SE	is calculated from the data.
(5)	S	is calculated from the parameters under H_A.

Note: This methodology will be employed to derive the sample size requirements for clinical trials, analyzed via censored survival analysis.

A136. THE POISSON PROCESS

INTRODUCTION

The Poisson Arrival Process is a logical model for patient accrual. The arrival rate (accrual rate), A, represents the expected number of patients to be accrued per unit time. The number of patients accrued in t units of time has a Poisson Distribution, with mean (At). Finally, conditional on the accrual of exactly n patients to time t, the n accrual times are uniformly distributed over the interval from 0 to t.

This will be an appropriate model for the accrual process of many clinical trials. First, there is a time scale, denoted by t. The Poisson process is simply a count N(t) of the number of patient entries up to time t.

Let us assume that we have a very large population of K patients. Assume that for a small interval of time of length Δt that the number of entries is binomial with sample size K and probability of incidence of disease

$$\frac{A\Delta t}{K}.$$

That is, the expected number of entries is $A\Delta t$, which is proportional to the length of Δt.

A137 <u>A is called the arrival rate or accrual rate</u>

We shall further assume that the number of entries in non-overlapping intervals are independent events. This may seem artificial, but is generally a reasonable assumption. The number of patients who develop the disease and leave the population will be a negligible fraction of K. The net effect of other departures and arrivals will also generally be a negligible fraction of K.

PLAN OF DERIVATION OF PROPERTIES

A138 (1) Divide the time scale from 0 to t into M intervals

$$0,\ \Delta t,\ 2\Delta t,\ \ldots,\ M\Delta t = T \qquad M = T/\Delta t.$$

A139 (2) Prove that as $K \to \infty$ and $\Delta t \to 0$ the probability that every interval has no more than one arrival goes to one. Hence, we can consider (in the limit) that each interval will have either 0 or 1 arrival.

A140 (3) Prove that as $K \to \infty$ and $\Delta t \to 0$

$$P\left[N(t) = x\right] \to (At)^x e^{-At}/x! \qquad x = 0, 1, \ldots$$

that is, $N(t)$ is Poisson with mean At.

A141 (4) Prove that the waiting time between arrivals is exponential with parameter A.

A142 (5) Suppose we have a Poisson Process (with arrival rate A) where arrivals are assigned by independent flips of a fair coin to treatment 1 and treatment 2. Then the two processes $N_1(t)$, the number of patients assigned to Treatment 1 by time t and $N_2(t)$, the number of patients assigned to Treatment 2 by time t are independent Poisson Processes with common arrival rates A/2.

A143 (6) In a Poisson process, given that r entries occur by time t, the entry times are uniformly distributed over the time interval from zero to t.

Proofs:

Prior to proving the results, two lemmas will be derived for later use.

A144 Lemma A:

Let $0 < |y| < 1$. Then there exists $z : |z| \leq |y|$ and $\log(1+y) = y - \frac{y^2}{2(1+z)^2}$

Proof: This is simply Taylor's Theorem applied to the second derivative

$$f(y) = \log(1+y) \qquad f(0) = 0$$

$$f'(y) = \frac{1}{1+y} \qquad f'(0) = 1$$

$$f''(y) = \frac{-1}{(1+y)^2}$$

Taylor's theorem states that there exists a $z : |z| \leq |y|$ with

$$f(y) = f(0) + yf'(0) + \frac{y^2}{2}f''(z)$$

A145 Lemma B:

Let $A_n \to \infty$ and $B_n \to \infty$ with $\frac{A_n}{B_n} \to 1$ as $n \to \infty$

$$W_n = \left(1 + \frac{x}{B_n}\right)^{A_n} \to e^x \text{ as } n \to \infty.$$

Proof: Since $B_n \to \infty$, there exists N such that whenever $n>N$, $|x/B_n| < \frac{1}{2}$. We shall work exclusively with $n>N$ so that logs are defined, and x/B_n is bounded away from -1.

Let $Y_n = \log W_n = A_n \log(1 + \frac{x}{B_n})$.

From Lemma A (A144), there exists $z_n : |z_n| \leq |x/B_n|$

$$Y_n = \frac{A_n x}{B_n} - \frac{A_n x^2}{2B_n^2(1+z_n)^2}. \qquad (*)$$

$$\frac{A_n x}{B_n} \to x \qquad \text{since } A_n/B_n \to 1$$

We show that second term of $(*)$ goes to zero.

Recall that $B_n \to \infty$ and $A_n/B_n \to 1$. Hence

$$0 < \frac{A_n x^2}{B_n^2(1+z_n)^2} \leq \frac{4}{B_n}\left(\frac{A_n}{B_n}\right) x^2 \to 0,$$

which implies

$$\frac{A_n x^2}{2B_n^2(1+z_n)^2} \to 0.$$

That is,

$$Y_n = \log(W_n) \to x.$$

That is $\quad W_n = e^{Y_n} \to e^x.$

We now return to the major derivation of results.

Proofs: (Main results)

First, we shall prove (2), that in the limit, multiple entries in any interval become impossible.

For a given interval, the probability of zero or one entry is obtained from the binomial distribution as

$$C = \left(1 - \frac{A\Delta t}{K}\right)^{K} + \frac{KA\Delta t}{K}\left(1 - \frac{A\Delta t}{K}\right)^{K-1} \qquad \text{(See A136)}$$

$$= \left(1 - \frac{A\Delta t}{K}\right)^{K-1}\left\{1 - \frac{A\Delta t}{K} + \frac{KA\Delta t}{K}\right\}$$

$$= \left(1 - \frac{A\Delta t}{K}\right)^{K-1}\left\{1 + \left(\frac{K-1}{K}\right) A\Delta t\right\}.$$

By independence, the probability of 0 or 1 entry in all M intervals is

$$C^M = \left(1 - \frac{A\Delta t}{K}\right)^{M(K-1)}\left\{1 + \left(\frac{K-1}{K}\right) A\Delta t\right\}^M.$$

Now $\Delta t = T/M$ and hence

$$C^M = \left(1 - \frac{AT}{MK}\right)^{M(K-1)}\left\{1 + \frac{(K-1)}{KM} AT\right\}^M$$

We apply Lemma B to each term

$$\left(1 - \frac{AT}{KM}\right)^{M(K-1)} \rightarrow e^{-AT}$$

Since M(K-1) and $MK \to \infty$ with $\frac{M(K\text{-}1)}{MK} \to 1.$

Also

$$\left\{1 + \frac{(K\text{-}1)AT}{KM}\right\}^M \to e^{AT}$$

since $M \to \infty$, $\frac{KM}{(K\text{-}1)} \to \infty$ with $\frac{M(K\text{-}1)}{KM} \to 1.$

That is, $C^M \to e^{-AT}e^{AT} = 1$. Thus (2) holds.

In the limit, we can ignore the possibility of multiple arrivals. This will help prove (3).

The probability of zero and one arrivals respectively in a single interval are

$$P_0 = \left(1 - \frac{A\Delta t}{K}\right)^K \text{ and } P_1 = A\Delta t\left(1 - \frac{A\Delta t}{K}\right)^{K-1}.$$

The probability of r arrivals to time t is simply binomial

$$D_r = \binom{M}{r} P_0^{M-r} P_1^r$$

$$= \binom{M}{r}\left(1 - \frac{A\Delta t}{K}\right)^{K(M-r)} (A\Delta t)^r \left(1 - \frac{A\Delta t}{K}\right)^{(K-1)r}$$

$$= \binom{M}{r}\left(1 - \frac{AT}{MK}\right)^{MK-r} \left(\frac{AT}{M}\right)^r \qquad (\Delta t = T/M)$$

$$= \left[\frac{M(M\text{-}1)(M\text{-}2)\cdots(M\text{-}r\text{+}1)}{M^r}\right]\frac{(At)^r}{r!}\left[1 - \frac{AT}{MK}\right]^{MK-r}. \qquad (**)$$

Now as $M \to \infty$, $K \to \infty$

$$\frac{M(M\text{-}1)\cdots(M\text{-}r\text{+}1)}{M^r} \to 1$$

and by Lemma B, and the fact that MK$\to\infty$ implies MK-r $\to \infty$ with (MK-r)/MK$\to$1,

$$\left[1 - \frac{AT}{MK}\right]^{MK-r} \to e^{-AT}.$$

That is, substituting in (**) the probability of r arrivals to time t,

$$D_r \to \frac{(AT)^r e^{-AT}}{r!}$$

This completes the proof of (3).

To prove (4), let us first look at the first arrival and show the time is exponential.

In order to have an arrival before time t, we must have $N(t) \geq 1$, that is, at least one arrival prior to time t.

$$\begin{aligned} P(\text{Arrival prior to time t}) &= P\Big((N(t) \geq 1\Big) \\ &= 1 - P\Big(N(t) = 0\Big) \\ &= 1 - (AT)^0 e^{-AT}/0! \\ &= 1 - e^{-At} \end{aligned}$$

The cumulative distribution of T_1, the time to the first arrival satisfies (see **A74**)

$$P\left[T_1 < t\right] = 1 - e^{-At} \qquad \text{(exponential)}$$

Now let T_r be the time of the rth arrival. From the independent interval binomial construction, the number of arrivals in the next t units of time, given T_r is Poisson with parameter At. $\Big(T_{r+1} - T_r$ is the time between the rth and $(r+1)^{th}$ arrival.$\Big)$

Hence

$$P\Big(T_{r+1} - T_r < t|T_r\Big) = P(\text{at least one arrival in t units of time})$$

$$= 1 - P(\text{no arrivals in t units of time})$$

$$= 1 - e^{At} \qquad \text{(exponential)}$$

This does not depend on T_r.

Hence, successive arrival times are independent identically distributed exponential random variables with parameter A.

To prove (5), it is clear from the structure discussed in **A136 - A138** that each of $N_1(t)$ and $N_2(t)$ is a Poisson Process with accrual rate (A/2). Further, the number of arrivals in a given interval to Treatment 1 and number of arrivals to a second interval (mutually exclusive of the first) are mutually independent events, since the overall process

$$N(t) = N_1(t) + N_2(t)$$

is constructed that way.

To complete the proofs, we need to show the somewhat surprising result that X_1, the number of patients assigned to Treatment 1 in a given interval is statistically independent of X_2, the number of patients assigned to Treatment 2 in the same interval.

Assuming the interval is of length t_1

$$P\left[X_1 = x_1, X_2 = x_2\right] = \frac{(At)^{x_1+x_2} e^{-At}}{(x_1+x_2)!} \binom{x_1+x_2}{x_1} (.5)^{x_1+x_2}$$

$$= \left[\frac{(At/2)^{x_1} e^{-At/2}}{x_1!}\right]\left[\frac{(At/2)^{x_2} e^{-At/2}}{x_2!}\right]$$

$$= P\left[X_1 = x_2\right] P\left[X_2 = x_2\right]$$

Hence X_1 and X_2 are independent as required.

Proof of (6)

Since successive arrival times are independent, identically distributed, exponential random variables, the joint distribution of the successive times between arrivals of the first (r+1) patients is

$$f(x_1, \ldots, x_{r+1}) = \prod_{j=1}^{r+1} \left(Ae^{-Ax_j}\right) \qquad \text{(exponential densities)}$$

$$= A^{r+1} e^{-A\sum_{j=1}^{r+1} x_j} \qquad x_1>0,\ x_2>0, \ldots$$

Note that this is only a function of

$$T_{r+1} = \sum_{j=1}^{r+1} x_j \text{ the total elapsed time until the } (r+1)^{st} \text{ arrival.}$$

Now we make a transformation (1-1)

$$T_1 = x_1$$

$$T_2 = x_1 + x_2$$

$$\vdots$$

$$T_r = x_1 + \cdots + x_r$$

$$T_{r+1} = (x_1 + x_2 + \cdots + x_{r+1}).$$

Since the Jacobian (see **A89** and **A90**), is unity,

the joint distribution of

$T_1, \ldots, T_{r+1}$ is

$$g(T_1, \ldots, T_{r+1}) = A^{r+1} e^{-AT_{r+1}} \qquad 0 < T_1 < T_2 < \cdots < T_{r+1}.$$

Let U be the event that exactly r arrivals have occurred by time t.

The conditional density of $(T_1, \ldots, T_r)$ given U is

$$g(T_1, \ldots, T_r | U) = \frac{\int_t^{\infty} g(T_1, \ldots, T_{r+1}) dT_{r+1}}{P(U)}.$$

Once the $T_1, \ldots, T_r$ with $T_r < t$ are fixed, U occurs only if $T_{r+1} > t$.

$$P(U) = P(\text{Exactly r arrivals to time t})$$

$$= \frac{(At)^r e^{-At}}{r!} \qquad \text{(Poisson Process).}$$

$$\int_t^\infty g(T_1, \ldots, T_{r+1})dT_{r+1} = A^{r+1}\int_t^\infty e^{-AT_{r+1}}dT_{r+1}$$

$$= A^r e^{-At}$$

Hence, the conditional density of $T_1, \ldots, T_r$ given U is

$$g(T_1, \ldots, T_r|U) = r!t^r \qquad 0 < T_1 < \cdots < T_r < t$$

That is, the ordered arrival times are uniformly distributed from zero to t. (This conditional density does not depend on the values of the T's provided they are ordered as above.)

This completes the discussion of the Poisson Process.

REFERENCES

1. **Fraser, D. A. S.,** *Probability and Statistics: Theory and Applications,* Duxbury Press, Boston, 1976.

2. **Hogg, R. V. and Craig, A. T.,** *Introduction to Mathematical Statistics,* Macmillan, New York, 1978.

3. **Mendenhall, W., Scheaffer, R. L., and Wackerly, D. D.,** *Mathematical Statistics with Applications,* Duxbury Press, Boston, 1986.

4. **Mood, A. M., Graybill, F. A., and Boes, D. C.,** *Introduction to the Theory of Statistics,* McGraw-Hill, New York, 1974.

5. **Suissa, S. and Shuster, J. J.,** Exact unconditional sample sizes for the 2 × 2 binomial trial, *J. R. Statist. Soc., Ser. A,* 148, 315, 1985.

INDEX

N

O

P

Q

R

S

T

U

V